THE
MAN
PLAN

JAMES TOOMBS MD

Disclaimer

The contents of this publication are intended to provide general information to a general public. The contents of this publication are no substitute for the medical diagnosis, advice or treatment from a licensed physician or other expert medical professional who personally examines you or your personal health information. All readers should seek personal consultation with and personal examination by a licensed physician or expert medical professional of their own choosing before commencing or adopting any exercise program, diet, or any other health-influencing practice for any general or specific health issue.

Author and publisher disclaim all responsibility for any liability, loss, or damage caused or alleged to be caused directly or indirectly as a consequence of the use, application or interpretation of the information in this publication.

ISBN: 1475067445
ISBN-13: 9781475067446
Library of Congress Control Number: 2012905508
CreateSpace, North Charleston, South Carolina

Acknowledgments

I owe sincere thanks to the following men who helped me transform some rambling thoughts into this book: Adam Bank, Jeff Fairbanks, Ian Fawks, Daniel Mattson and Steve Spencer. Their honest comments and critique were invaluable.

I also want to thank Victoria Skurnick for her guidance and assistance through the publication process.

Most of all, I want to thank my beautiful wife Celia for her infinite patience and support with this project.

James Toombs

Table of Contents

CHAPTER 1

Outrunning the Fat Man

_____

The sunlight filters through the leaves, casting shadows across my path. A gentle breeze brings the smell of the cool forest to me. It is late afternoon and I am hiking my favorite trail at a park near my home. There is a sharp snap of a twig behind me and I turn to see that I am not alone. I have no wish to share this time with anyone so I pick up my pace a little, just to put some distance between us. After a few minutes, I turn for a glance and see he has kept up with me. This trespasser looks familiar but no one I readily place. There is a small stab of anxiety and the worry "Am I being followed?" As I start to jog, to my surprise, he does, too. The fear factor starts creeping up my spine. I break into a run and the footsteps behind me follow suit. Now I am running full out wondering how this pale chubby man is keeping up and what his intentions might be. A glance over my shoulder and I see his arm reach for me. Then I wake up. Just a nightmare but I realize I am sweating and thirsty. In the bathroom, I grab my cup and switch on the light. I drop my cup as I look in the mirror and see the pale man. He is more than chubby, he is fat and flabby. And the worst: perched on his bulging belly are two man breasts.

Doctor, what does all this mean?

It is quite simple. You are in a modern day Dickens' tale and you have seen what you will become without an intervention. Now, let me show you the next chapter. . .

As a teenager, I was fit, trim and athletic. This was before the age of home computers, Playstations and 200 channels on cable TV. I spent little time sitting and studying. If not doing some random chore around the house, I was hiking or biking with my friends. While never a good athlete, I participated in high school sports ranging from wrestling to tennis. During the summer, I swam on the community pool's team. There was never a worry about my weight or health and I cannot recall ever giving a thought about food in terms of content or calories.

In contrast to high school, I had to study in college and also gave up team sports and any organized exercise program. All freshmen were sentenced to the dormitory for the first year. Eating a steady diet of dorm and junk food, the slim, muscular body I had in August was tarnished by May. In 9 months, I had put on the traditional "freshman fifteen." For the first time in my life, I had a belly. It was embarrassing when my little sister pointed it out. This should have been a warning to me. Over the summer, I started back jogging and the belly went away. When I returned to college the next fall, I took a class in weight lifting and also moved off campus, away from the endless buffet of food. My budget only allowed basic food stuffs, soups, sandwiches and such.

My major was geology and that was helpful for fitness. We spent a considerable time hiking the woods, mapping, investigating and collecting. In any aspect of life, including fitness, it helps to have a role model. Mine was my roommate. Mike was an NCAA track star and we both wore the same size shoes. He was sponsored by the Kangaroo Shoe Company and gifted me many pair. He also coached me directly and indirectly and I progressed from jogging to become a medium distance runner, 5-10 miles many days of the week. Through the rest of college, I was fit, trim and athletic.

After graduation my days changed materially. My first real job was behind a desk for a small actuarial firm. One particular benefit of the company was food. They provided donuts and pastries every morning along with a hot lunch at noon. Snacks, usually chips and candy bars, appeared in the early afternoon. This had the desired effect of keeping me at my desk working all day. I should also mention that with graduation, I gave up running and lifting. This combination, no exercise and no restraint, had the undesired effect of adding a very noticeable 25 pounds to my medium frame. Again, I had the belly, bigger than before. This should have been my second warning. Fortunately, I changed jobs after about a year, leaving the endless buffet behind. Adding running in the evenings helped wrangle my weight back into submission. In time, the belly was gone but so was a big part of my fitness edge.

Looking at family pictures, the belly is apparent in both my grandfathers. As they aged, it simply grew and grew. I have the belly gene. And so do you. It is a survival gene and brought our species through the famines of the centuries. It keeps us eating beyond satiety to pack on the requisite pounds to survive a cold foodless winter. Without the threat of starvation real and looming, the belly gene produces a survival disadvantage both in terms of health and fertility. For most Americans, food is now available in whatever variety we want and in whatever quantity we wish. We can simply choose to eat without end. The result is 70% of American males have a weight problem. The graph is based on CDC data, reflecting the percentage of Americans that are overweight, obese or extremely obese. Since 1960, it appears we have really made some progress.

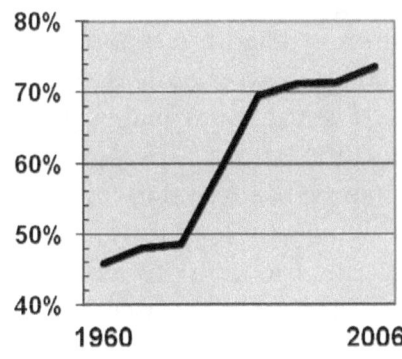

Another aspect of human life that has changed dramatically is work. Even in the recent past, most American males had physically demanding jobs in the fields and factories. The bicep and back have been replaced by tractors and robots. Now most of us find ourselves at desk jobs in some form or fashion. Our careers may be mentally challenging but the physical element of labor is missing. We rely solely on passive transportation and drive instead of walking or biking to the grocery store. We have stopped playing, too. Men have discarded physical leisure time activities like tennis and golf and the outlets for sedentary play at computers and televisions have only increased. More than 50% of the men in the U.S. do not get 10 minutes of vigorous physical activity a week. The National Institute of Health's definition of physical activity is pretty loose and includes anything that causes an increase in breathing or heart rate. Vacuuming and gardening are on the list. Even including trivial activities, most of us still get less than 10 minutes a week!

Increasing food along with decreasing physical activity. You could call this the perfect storm against manhood, but the combination of circumstances is not at all rare. As I age, is it my destiny to gain weight and lose muscle? Must I become fat and flabby? Do I have to grow man boobs? And along the way, am I slated to accumulate traditional man illnesses like high blood pressure, coronary artery disease, diabetes and erectile dysfunction?

Eventually, probably ten thousand years from now, I expect the belly gene will get turned off as obesity proves to be a powerful survival disadvantage. Quite simply, obese males will not be able to reproduce. Too obese to produce quality sperm. Too obese to have erections. Too far-fetched? Even now, the health consequences of obesity are affecting male fertility with 52% of obese men having fertility difficulties.

The risk of erectile dysfunction in obese males ranges as high as 90%. Certain undesirable genes, like the one causing Alzheimer's disease, stay in the gene pool because their effect occurs after reproductive age. Consider for a moment that obesity is taking hold of our children. Childhood obesity has tripled in the past 30 years and nearly 20% are now considered obese. Fertility issues will be impacting them soon if they have not already.

The term I have coined for this common male condition is the Fat Sedentary Lifestyle. In the remainder of the book, I will just abbreviate it FSL to help with clarity and brevity as we move forward. "Fat" refers to daily caloric excess, not simply weight, body structure or abdominal girth. In my context, it does not mean "obese." It simply means more calories are consumed than necessary to meet the body's current need. In time, it produces obesity. The "sedentary lifestyle" refers to anyone who spends most of their day on their butt or back with little or no vigorous physical exercise.

The body does not support something it does not use. Contrary to the popular belief, unused muscle does not turn to fat, it simply withers. The medical term for this is atrophy. With a proper exercise challenge, muscle cells respond and grow (hypertrophy). As with my case, weight gain in men may be fairly rapid when life circumstances change-college, work, marriage or divorce for example. Weight gain that accompanies aging is usually a slow, subtle process and typically begins in the early twenties. On average, men add just over two pounds per year. The 20 pounds you put on since college is not likely muscle. Body composition typically changes, too. Men tend to lose muscle mass at the rate of one percent per year. A two pound gain likely represents losing one pound of muscle and adding three pounds of fat.

What about the man boobs? Are they a guarantee? Absolutely not. Genes are the architect's building plans but along the way they are influenced by the environment, activity and access to materials. Even a detailed building plan does not guarantee a particular outcome. The human building plan has plenty of adaptability built in. With regards to work and food, our situation has changed more quickly than certain genes can be deactivated. Understanding how to manage them is the foundation of the Man Plan.

In 1996, my actuarial career went careening off the beaten path and I entered medical school. At age 33, I was the oldest student in my class of 96. To this point in my life, fitness was more like an event than a lifestyle. Something that you gained then lost. I got the final push to stay permanently fit as I neared the end of my training. Following medical school and residency, prior to entering practice, I elected to complete a pain medicine fellowship. It was about six months before graduation when I received a notice from the Army. I would be headed to Iraq in the fall of 2004. Damn! In medical school, I was in very good shape. I ran almost every day, five to seven miles, and did a marathon (or ultra marathon) once or twice a year. In addition to time, I had an exceptional motivator in the form of an exceptional running partner. Medical school was busy but I still made enough time to run.

That precious commodity evaporated in residency. We were "limited" to working just 80 hours per week. That still left 88 hours of personal time for eating, sleeping, studying, home and family. The 80 hour work week came in the form of long days and overnight shifts. Neither was conductive to regular exercise. In retrospect, I could have worked out and I might have had a better attitude and more energy for it. Instead, I exercised too little and, again, ate too much. When I started fellowship, I weighed 25 pounds more than

I did in medical school. How many times will I gain and lose this same 25 pounds? More important than my actual weight was my body composition. I went from 10% body fat to 22%.

I was thankful for the advanced warning about my deployment. It gave me six months to lose 25 lbs. Simple, I thought "I'll just start working out again." My initial program was jogging 20-30 minutes three times a week. And after a month, there was no change in my weight. I could not even say my pants fit better. So I started lifting weights on the days I was not jogging. And after another month, still no change in weight. Had I become someone who just couldn't lose weight? I was getting concerned that I would not be in shape for deployment. Yes, I would be going to Iraq as a doctor but in 2004, Iraq was still a shooting war and doctors were expected to move out with the troops.

With four months before I shipped overseas, I started to focus on my diet. In fellowship, we had an endless buffet of food at the hospital and I took advantage of it. It was some poor consolation for the long hours of work. This had to go. I started eating breakfast at home, taking my lunch and healthy snacks. To this point in my life, only minimal changes were necessary to get back in shape. That is the benefit of youth. After age 40, I discovered that diet changes, mostly eating less, are a central element in losing weight. In month 3, my jogging returned to running and my toning program at the gym became true weight lifting. The weight finally started to come off. Over the next 3 months, I lost 25 pounds. My focus then was clearly more on weight loss than building muscle but I did gain a fair amount of strength, too.

Ron White, one of my favorite comedians, has an exceptional joke about Anecdote and Antidote and how close the words sound but how different their meanings are. His joke is about a snake bite and how someone would have lived if he had known the difference. In fitness, can you spot the difference? An antidote by definition is a remedy or agent used to counteract the effects of a poison. In health and fitness, we want the antidote but get anecdotes. On television and in the press, we get tips and trivia about exercise, weight loss and health. The format of many fitness magazines is little more than a series of training anecdotes and some are endless advertisements for weightlifting supplements. I called this book the Man Plan. In reality, I could have called it Man's Antidote. The toxic agent is the FSL. It induces a progressive feminization and, in time, it will emasculate you. The elements that steal your manhood, obesity and inactivity, can be counteracted, overpowered and defeated at any point. In my own program, I made the training mistakes of an amateur. You could follow the same twisted trail. Or you could be educated and efficient. The Man Plan is about education and efficiency.

Obesity is an epidemic in the United States and accounts for an estimated 300,000 deaths per year. Because it poses such a significant health risk, it is well studied with a vast amount of information available. Exercise is well researched too, though often in smaller more focused studies. The crux of the problem is how to get to the information that is accurate and practical. Many fitness tales are repeated until they become truth. When I began my own program, I subscribed to several fitness magazines but the tips and techniques were a jumble of information. Some of the information, even within a single issue was conflicting. Many of the tips were suitable for an advanced lifter: How to change the shape of your bicep. I wanted to change the shape of my entire body.

I made it to age 40 without a concrete plan on how to maintain a man shape and I am a doctor. In retrospect, I got back into shape almost by accident. Along the way, I made every beginner mistake. I overestimated the caloric value of jogging and weight lifting and underestimated the impact of my eating habits. It is very comforting to have a huge sundae after being on call overnight. Through trial and error and more error, I did get fit, mostly because of the deployment lurking in the shadows. In Iraq, I lifted or ran almost every day. Returning to the U.S., I stuck with it. For a period, my program remained old school, lots of time in the gym. In college and medical school, with surplus time, it was feasible option. Now with a family, career and second job, too, it had to change. The Army battle plan changed with Desert Storm and the wars in Iraq and Afghanistan. Rather than pouring it on, combat is about efficiency, the right force directed at the problem. When you spend your energies fighting the FSL you want progress. I wanted to figure out not just how to do it but how to do it efficiently. The goal was to apply the right forces and not spend three hours a day at the gym. I simply did not have that kind of time. That led to questions. As I started learning more, the time I spent in the gym and on the track dropped but my lean body mass, strength and speed kept increasing. Fitness is a dose response curve, more is better. But better is better, too.

While researching I came upon various books and articles equivalent to "How to get fit in 10 minutes a day." If this were true, obesity in the United States would end as we know it. Who would not invest 10 minutes a day to look like Lance Armstrong? What the authors appeared to be measuring was the improvement from doing absolutely nothing physical during the day to doing something physical for 10 solid minutes. And to a degree, it works, but only to a degree. The theory behind 10-minutes-a-day fitness is simple: A poor plan is better than no plan. I disagree entirely. I think a poor plan can be reinforcing to the idea that change is impossible. When you find that you are not making any significant progress, you begin believing that you are someone who cannot lose weight or get fit. I had an overwhelming need to become fit and kept pushing. Without that, I am not sure I would have continued my efforts given my initial failures.

In writing this book, I have utilized the wealth of resources available through PubMed. This is a free database with access to more than 20 million citations for biomedical literature from MEDLINE, life science journals and online books. It is maintained by the United States National Library of Medicine and the National Institutes of Health. I have taken formal medical research and placed it in a practical context. If you read this book cover-to-cover, you will have more information concerning health and exercise physiology than I learned in medical school, residency and fellowship combined. You may want a medical dictionary handy, too. There is no spoon feeding here.

There are no miracles presented, but there may be surprises. If you methodically put these principles into practice, you will be successful. The hardest part is getting started. If you are reading this book, you have made the first step in your own Man Plan. Within the pages, I hope you will find that one element that pushes you to action. Once you commit to your program, it will become easier. Progress breeds more progress. It is in our souls to compete, even with ourselves. I find myself continually setting challenges and markers. The whys and hows you can gain from reading, but you have to commit the wheres and whens. The Man Plan is a way of life, not an event.

From a physician's perspective, why you should exercise is an easy question to answer. Why you start exercising boils down to a simple question, too. Do you want to stay a man?

CHAPTER 2

The Factory

———

Let me open with an apology. This chapter is about physiology, necessary background but fairly dry. It is an essential chapter to describe the key players and health outcomes related to the FSL. There are few opportunities for dick jokes, but I will get back to them in the next section. In terms of information content, these brief remarks are more up-to-date than my 1996 physiology text. Over the past 15 years, as the obesity epidemic has raged, the number of medical studies regarding fat metabolism has exploded, too. Unfortunately, "understanding" has not translated into "changing." Without a magic anti-fat pill, we must rely on our superior intellect to thrash our lagging genes.

Our relationship with fat begins before birth. The last month of pregnancy is for gaining weight, about ½ pound a week. Fat is packed on so we can survive until our ability to consume calories increases. At birth, an infant's body is 25% fat on average. The very act of eating is fatiguing for infants; food must be efficient. Through breast milk, babies receive about 40% of their calories from fat and this is processed quite easily with more than 95% of the calories available for energy. In contrast, the cost to process carbohydrates is about 30% of the calories consumed. Nearly 80% of the calories expended by a neonate are for regulation of body temperature and development. Less than 10% are expended in activity. A baby gaining weight is getting enough calories. After infancy, humans enter the leanest period of their lives and do not rebound until age five.

Fat on the human body is organized into three general types: brown, subcutaneous and visceral. Brown fat is specialized for producing heat and neonates are born with a fair percentage of it. This helps maintain body temperature in infants and virtually disappears with time. Only a trivial amount remains in adults in the neck and upper back. Just under the skin is subcutaneous fat. If you have ever had a deep cut, or watched liposuction on reality television, you may have seen the glistening yellow globs. Subcutaneous fat covers the body in a near continuous sheet, giving us not only energy storage but insulation. It thickens the skin and gives women their decorative curves, boobs and buns. When men pack on fat, we get the same curves and the bonus belly. Subcutaneous fat can be removed by the pound with liposuction or returned by the ounce through injection, usually in the face to replace aging losses. Visceral fat is found throughout the intraabdominal cavity. Kidneys are padded with mounds of visceral fat and sheets of it, the mesentery and omentum, surround the intestines.

Both subcutaneous and visceral fat are huge reservoirs of energy. The average 200 pound man has enough stored power in fat to run just over 900 miles. Each fat cell contains a small control center, the nucleus. This is flattened to the side by a semi-liquid droplet of fat contained within the cell. Excess calories are stored first subcutaneously and as this reservoir nears capacity, fat is packed on viscerally. The relative accumulation of subcutaneous to visceral fat is inherited. Babies are born with a moderate number of fat cells. Gradually, the number of cells increase and are generally set by adolescence. But fat capacity is only a relative term. If we need more space for fat storage, the cells first increase in size (hypertrophy) before they divide and increase in number (hyperplasia). When we lose weight, the cells do not completely disappear; they only shrink, waiting to be refilled.

Historically, fat had been considered fairly inert, literally, hanging around to be used up during the cold winter. The belly is more like a cashier's drawer than a bank vault and there is a constant exchange with the blood stream. Two key hormones, insulin and glucagon, guide this process. When we eat, insulin is released from the pancreas and directs the liver, muscles and fat cells to take up glucose for storage. Insulin also halts the use of fat for energy. Low blood glucose triggers the release of glucagon which, in turn, indirectly signals for the breakdown of fat for energy. For survival, men must maintain a minimum quantity of body fat, about 2-4 percent. The average man these days is about 25 percent body fat. If his body weight is 200 pounds, he has 50 pounds of pure fat tucked under his skin and in his belly. The fat on his body weighs more than his brain, heart, liver and kidneys, combined. In recent years, science has discovered that fat is anything but lazy. It turns out visceral fat is a major endocrine organ releasing a host of chemical signals into the blood stream. Fat is a factory producing adiponectin, resistin, plasminogen activator inhibitor-1, tumor necrosis factor-alpha (TNFα), interleukin-6, and leptin. Wow! Each one in the category of "Things I forgot after medical school." All of them have an important role in the normal function and maintenance of the human body. As visceral fat grows, some of these chemicals increase in concentration and, paradoxically, others drop.

The earliest humans had to scramble for food; our genetic push was toward obesity. This ability to store energy efficiently as fat has been a grand success story. Man, like most animals, has internal controls for metabolism. There is synchronization between activity, weight and appetite.

In the past 100 years, human physical activity levels have dramatically dropped. We have compensated and our food intake has been trimmed. Despite having a buffet laid before us every day, we pretty much stay in caloric balance. Eating turns off the appetite and it works nearly perfectly. Nearly. Over the course of 10 years, the usual male adds twenty pounds. Given there are about 72,000 calories in twenty pounds fat and 3650 days in that same period, the average male is only out of balance by 19.72 calories per day. That is one bite of a chocolate brownie. Why our bodies are not in perfect caloric balance is an unsettled medical debate that rages. One conclusion is our genes never anticipated encountering the endless buffet we now have and, therefore, no biological countermeasures exists. Some researchers are convinced we are simply not equipped to deal with the glucose spikes of refined sugars and high fructose corn syrup. The rapid introduction of high glycemic index and processed foods into the human diet has neatly overwhelmed the control systems.

The light bulb may share some of the blame. With the invention of electric lighting, our sleep patterns have changed dramatically. Sleep is window for rejuvenation of the body's systems. During sleep, growth hormone is released and cortisol, our stress hormone is inhibited. Adults need eight or more hours a night; most get far less. More of our work is knowledge based not physical. While sleep and cognitive work are both sedentary activities, they have opposite effects on appetite. Sleep normalizes appetite whereas desk work increases it. Understanding this, gave me an explanation of why I had such trouble maintaining weight in residency and fellowship, eating more is a natural consequence of not getting enough sleep. What drove my first employer to provide food all day long? Were they merely feeding the desires of deskbound workers or was it something more sinister? Watching television is another "activity" that increases the intake of calorie dense foods; obesity can be correlated directly with hours spent in front of the TV.

A number of experts claim that obesity is just an obvious state of fat overload and attribute the ill health effects on the accumulation of lipid metabolites in the tissues. While we can study the individual effects of hormones, metabolites, sleep and activity, it quickly becomes the story of the blind men describing an elephant by feeling the trunk, tail or tusk. Each study may have some truth to it; the entire picture is not yet clear. Genetically and environmentally, we remain very susceptible to getting fat.

While we wait on the full explanation of "why" there are a number of observations that can be related. In a man's life there is a tipping point regarding the loss of metabolic control. It occurs predictably with the right combination of age, increased body fat and low physical activity. With aging, growth hormone drops. The belly is a combination of subcutaneous and visceral fat. With a fall in growth hormone, subcutaneous fat migrates, in a fashion, to become visceral fat. Without gaining an ounce, men can gain a paunch and the factory that comes with it. When visceral fat reaches a critical mass, it exerts significant influence on the body. The net effect is not normalization but acceleration. Essentially, the bus is going too fast so the driver presses on the gas pedal.

As we eat, insulin levels increase, signaling the liver, muscles and fat cells to begin uptake of glucose and store energy. With belly fat, there is resistance to the effects of insulin, called appropriately, insulin resistance. Although the association is clear, the exact cause remains uncertain. Leptin is the chemical signal related to satiety, the feeling of satisfied fullness. Normally, the decline in circulating leptin signals impending starvation. Eating restores the leptin levels and hunger is satisfied. This is the very definition of feedback control. However, the belly elevates leptin levels and through the process, we lose control of our appetite. Adiponectin released by visceral fat decreases in obesity and sensitivity of muscles to insulin is lost. These three signals, insulin, leptin and adiponectin, swirl in a vicious cycle, further escalating obesity. The result is called "metabolic syndrome."

Medically speaking, syndromes are a work in progress, similar to an aircraft accident investigation. We comb through the wreckage, looking for clues but the precise cause may remain elusive. More often than not, crashes are an intersection of multiple factors. For the time being, metabolic syndrome is a description of facts and circumstances, not a diagnosis. It is clearly a combination of factors. Nearly all patients with metabolic syndrome are a little older and all have adopted the FSL. Along with increased belly fat, we see elevated triglycerides, decreased HDL cholesterol (the good kind), increased blood pressure and insulin resistance expressed as increased fasting glucose. Youth is somewhat protective and exercise can help normalize insulin resistance but fails to provide complete protection. College football linemen are the largest players on the field, relying on size and explosive strength. Despite vigorous workouts, when linemen reach a certain level of body fat, they start showing the signs and symptoms of metabolic syndrome. In a study of college lineman, nearly 60% had metabolic syndrome. There are also men with a falsely reassuring "normal" body weight with metabolic syndrome. They may not have gained a pound since college but their body composition has certainly changed. The loss of muscle and the accumulation of belly fat have simply matched each other.

With the subtle accumulation of visceral fat, they get metabolic syndrome, too.

The health effects of metabolic syndrome are far reaching and associated with a host of medical conditions. Science cannot emphatically state that metabolic syndrome causes any of them, it only increases the risk. It is akin to driving down the highway at ninety miles an hour. You may not get a speeding ticket. You may not have an accident. Nonetheless, the risk that either might happen goes up dramatically. Metabolic syndrome is most closely associated with Type II diabetes and heart disease. Insulin resistance associated with metabolic syndrome may give rise to Type II diabetes, requiring medications or insulin to control blood sugars. High triglycerides and low HDL cholesterol are key risk factors for heart disease. Add in a little high blood pressure and you have the recipe for a heart attack.

The health risk from the FSL is not just from metabolic syndrome. With obesity, all-cause mortality increases. Simply stated: obesity increases the death rate by at least 20% and may increase it as high as 200% in the morbidly obese. As I remarked earlier, fat is a factory. Two of the products of belly fat, tumor necrosis factor-alpha (TNFα) and interleukin-1, are inflammatory mediators. Their release may lead to a state of chronic inflammation and the very mechanisms used to protect against infection are turned against the body. Inflammation can cause damage to the lining of arteries, the endothelium, sparking atherosclerosis and clogged arteries. The promotion of atherosclerosis by belly fat is independent of age. In a large percentage of American men, the first symptom of coronary artery disease is merely sudden death.

Not worried about heart disease? How about stroke? High blood pressure is one risk factor, atherosclerosis is another. Clots can form in the brain's own blood supply or travel from elsewhere and clog an artery. A substance called tissue plasminogen activator (tPA) helps break up clots that form in the body giving us some protection. Doctors even treat strokes by administering a clone of tPA within the small window of time before brain tissue has died. How does fat cause a stroke? Belly fat produces tPA's antagonist, plasminogen activator inhibitor-1, a substance that prevents the breakdown of blood clots. Without it the clot remains and the stroke is completed.

Obesity and belly fat are associated with an increased risk of all types of cancer including: colon, kidney, pancreas, prostate and stomach. It is not clear if this is related to exaggerated cell division or from the loss of immune functions that could destroy cancerous cells at the outset.

The physical state of obesity can overstress bones and joints. A pound on the belly applies a force of 5-6 pounds across the knee hastening the breakdown of cartilage. There is more to the picture than mechanical stress; the inflammatory chemicals released by visceral fat, seem to play a role in arthritis overall. Belly weight changes the geometry of the normal back, increasing anterior pelvic tilt, reducing range of motion and accelerating the disc degeneration shown on magnetic resonance imaging (MRI). Pregnant women universally develop back pain. The "persistent pregnancy" of an obese male can have the same effect.

Breathing seems to be an essential element of life. Obesity can bring on a condition called sleep apnea. Essentially, you stop breathing briefly while you sleep. With each stop, the oxygen saturation in the blood drops and this can ultimately lead to heart failure. Muscle tone normally relaxes during sleep but with obesity, fat deposits in the neck complement the relaxation and cause a mechanical collapse of the airway during sleep. Equally important are the chemicals released by visceral fat. These may cause central nervous system depression and a loss of neuromuscular control in the upper airway. The rub is this: obesity causes sleep apnea which, in turn, worsens obesity which in turn, worsens sleep apnea. Another vicious obesity cycle.

Did I mention that both kidney stones and gallstones are increased in obesity? They are. Are there any health benefits to being fat? What about fat men being jolly? Remember Santa Claus? Nope. Obesity is also linked to depression and other mood disorders.

Is there a good word in any of this? Well, not really, except now you have the essence of a thousand studies confirming the belly is more than a decoration and the FSL is not a harmless vice. Having a belly puts your life at risk in any number of ways. This entire chapter could have been shortened to "The FSL is really, really bad for you" but that does not appeal to the adult learners need for relevance and reason. The past few paragraphs detail the lion's share of recognized, significant and largely unspoken consequences of the FSL. By continuing the FSL, you have given informed consent for all harm that might follow. You are solely responsible for the butcher's bill. Beware, the butcher is eyeing your manhood, too.

CHAPTER 3

Progressive Feminization

———

Where would we be without testosterone? Frankly, we would all be women. In humans, female is the default sex and without testosterone, you get ovaries and a vagina. Mom gave us the X chromosome but our lives as men begin with a gift from our father, the Y chromosome. Up to about week 7, embryos are gonadally identical; the sex of a fetus cannot be determined with an ultrasound peek. On this blessed Y chromosome, there is a small, small section that codes for testis determining factor (TDF). This protein acts on the undifferentiated gonads and guides their development. The primary sex cords become seminiferous tubules and the testicle forms. The names of body parts almost always have their roots in Latin or Greek. Regarding testicle, there is no consensus on how this term was derived. In Latin, the word testis meant witness. Are testicles, then, the witness of masculinity and virility?

With TDF, the little gonads have a full set of marching orders and, by week 8, they start their lifetime of work. An initial item of business for the new testicle is producing mullerian inhibiting substance (MIS). This actively halts female development, preventing the growth of a uterus, an unnecessary anatomic accessory for men. At least until puberty, the principal testicular product, of course, is testosterone. Men and women have complementary parts. Under the influence of testosterone, the undifferentiated external genitalia begin to take shape, literally. The embryonic phallus lengthens becoming the penis, not the clitoris. Folds of labioscrotal tissue, aptly named, fuse to form the scrotum. The testicles, developing in the abdomen, begin their trek south and enter the scrotum near 28 weeks. By birth, our small man parts are complete and we emerge identifiable as little boys.

The male sex hormone has been extracted from various animal testicles for the past hundred years. In 1935, it was finally isolated in a fair quantity and given a name, testosterone, a combination of three words: testes, steroid and ketone. Humbly beginning as cholesterol, testosterone becomes a steroid hormone in a short biosynthetic pathway. The chemical formula, $C_{19}H_{28}O_2$, is below:

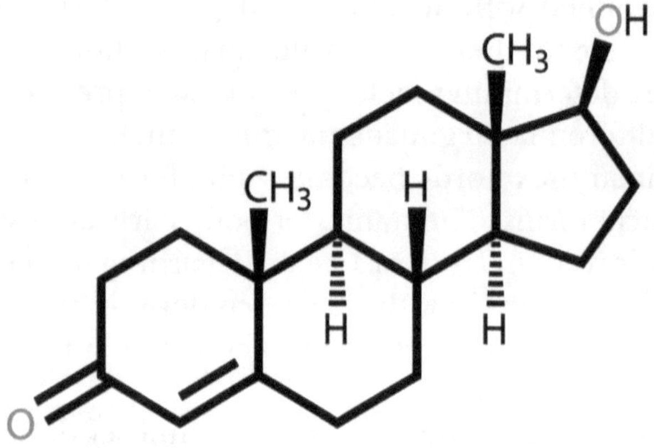

Testosterone is quite powerful stuff and the driver of a man's nitrogen balance. Most nitrogen in the body is part of protein. A positive nitrogen balance, where more is retained than excreted, means muscle growth. At certain levels testosterone will produce muscular development without exercise. One study discovered men treated with testosterone gained more than 4 pounds of lean tissue despite being at complete bed rest for 28 days.

There is a very close relationship of testosterone with estradiol, a female sex hormone. Estradiol is just one step further down a chemical pathway and the compounds differ by only a methyl and carbonyl group. Chemically, they are nearly identical but distinct enough to stimulate different hormone receptors. The conversion of testosterone to estrogen is completed via an aromatase, an enzyme found principally in fat. This reaction made perfect sense to me in organic chemistry and now I understand the application. In normal healthy men, estrogen has a function and there is a small amount of aromatase present to meet this need. With some ominous foreshadowing, I will simply state that too much aromatase will produce too much estrogen.

After birth, testosterone levels rise briefly, and then drop back to nearly undetectable levels. No apparent physical changes can be attributed to testosterone during this window. There is a belief that it plays a role in masculinization of the brain. Through adolescence, testosterone is only a minor player. With puberty, however, the Leydig cells in the testicles begin churning out testosterone. The testicles grow and move away from the body acquiring the necessary sag to stay a few degrees cooler, a requirement for developing sperm. The penis, not having changed much in size or shape since infancy, begins to lengthen and take on an adult form.

During puberty and early adulthood, the blood level of testosterone increases like wild fire and we reap the benefits of this hormonal storm. In addition to the physical changes to our man equipment, nearly every other body system is affected. Testosterone is responsible for bone structure, giving men broad shoulders and a narrow waist. It accounts for our muscle bulk, fat distribution and body hair. It lengthens the vocal cords, deepens the voice and constructs the Adam's apple. Testosterone is responsible for all aspects of fertility. It directs the Sertoli cells in the testicles to produce sperm and gives us sex drive and erections. Development into manhood is directly dependent on the level of circulating testosterone. Maintenance of these same qualities remains dependent on a continuing supply of circulating testosterone. Simply stated: If you were born with a penis, you must have testosterone to keep it.

Secretion of testosterone is controlled by hormones released from the brain: gonadotropin releasing hormone (GnRH) from the hypothalamus and luteinizing hormone (LH) from the pituitary. Negative feedback controls keep it in check. There is a wide range of testosterone levels in men; a healthy normal is somewhere 350 and 1200 measured in nanograms per deciliter of blood. Overall, 70% of testosterone in the blood is bound to sex hormone-binding globulin (SHBG) leaving just 30% biologically available as free testosterone. The testicles have no testosterone storage capacity. Blood concentration follows a circadian rhythm in younger men, typically spiking in the morning, after a good night's sleep. This accounts for morning wood. The spikes flatten with age and may not follow any particular pattern. After a peak in the late teens or early twenties, testosterone level typically begins a slow progressive decline, about 1% per year. However, not all men become deficient as they age. That begs the question regarding cause and consequence.

Ovaries have an abbreviated life; they start failing in a woman's late forties and, on average, quit entirely at age fifty-one. No more eggs, no more estrogen. In stark contrast, a man can produce sperm and testosterone until the day he dies (hopefully, while having sex!). A man's testosterone level and testicular function are determined by a complex interaction of genetic, environmental, and even societal factors. Genetics determine our individual basal testosterone level. Men have a large capacity to steer this up or down, depending on our choices. Specific elements like a good night's sleep and appropriate diet can boost testosterone. On the other hand, the FSL drives testosterone levels into the ground through the reciprocal interactions of decreased production and increased conversion. When we chose a sedentary life, the testosterone factory slows considerably and basal levels begin to drop. Fat is the largest source of aromatase in both males and females, and this enzyme actively converts circulating testosterone to estrogen. Increasing parallel to estrogen is SHBG, which further decreases free and biologically available testosterone. More E and less free T. This is a goal for male-to-female transsexuals but an unintentional outcome of the FSL.

For men, just a whiff of estrogen is necessary for "bone" maintenance. With the FSL, we get more than bones, we get man boobs. The medical term, gynecomastia, is the proliferation of male breast tissue. While certain medications might cause it, male breast enlargement is most frequently linked to increased estrogen and decreased testosterone. With the FSL, part of these chest decorations may be actual breast tissue, but, for the most part, they are simple fat. The growth of breasts should be a warning shout to any man, "You have too much estrogen." A glance in the mirror can tell you as much as a blood test. It is an unmistakable reflection of the progressive feminization that occurs with the FSL.

Smoking clearly has many significant long-term health effects. As 90% of those who die from smoking start before age eighteen, there is a serious effort to dissuade teens from picking up the habit. Numerous information-based interventions have failed to reveal an effective tactic. The potential physical costs of smoking, emphysema, heart disease, and lung cancer, are so far in the future, they are universally discounted by the youthful smoker. Smoking also damages the collagen fibers in the skin that give it strength and elasticity. These changes happen in as little as ten years and are irreversible. One group of researchers studying young female smokers applied aging software to current photographs. When smoking related changes were added, the effect was quite powerful, motivating many to consider quitting. Young women recognizing this single obvious physical change related to smoking became concerned about losing that glowing beacon of youth and femininity, their face. Likewise, a man's body is the trophy he carries everywhere. The FSL destroys this monument and builds a self-sustaining estrogen factory. The most effective image to convince a man to reject the FSL may be man boobs.

If only it were boobs, the FSL might be a tolerable compromise, after all, I do like eating and TV. Unfortunately, man boobs are just the introduction; the rest of the story is much worse. While the boobs are growing, the FSL is silently eroding the very foundation of manhood. Metabolic syndrome, diabetes, and obesity are all associated with hypogonadism, the medical term for underperforming testicles. More painfully descriptive terms might be small, shrunken, or withered. There is no precise explanation for the cause, but it relates to levels of leptin, luteinizing hormone, insulin, and estrogen, among others. The brain basically slows in sending hormonal signals to the testicles. One study noted that 12% of patients with metabolic syndrome had hypogonadism regardless of age. This compares to 4% in the healthy population. With diabetes, low testosterone occurs in 40% of men age forty. Compare that figure to healthy eighty-year-old men where only 20% have low testosterone.

Obesity without diabetes is no safe haven. Four out of ten obese men over age forty-five have hypogonadism. There is positive feedback between hypogonadism and obesity. Low testosterone predisposes fat accumulation, and fat suppresses testosterone production, a vicious cycle. The combination of diabetes and obesity is even more destructive, where fully half have low testosterone.

So my testosterone is low and I've grown boobs, at least I can still have sex. Well, maybe not. Testosterone is a cruel mistress. It only takes a hint of T to want sex, but a firm penis involves a whole lot more. Erections are a masterpiece of engineering, a complex process involving desires, hormones, nerves, arteries, and spongy tissues in the penis. With the right input—sight, smell, touch—nerves give autonomic signals to the small penile arteries. They dilate, allowing erectile tissue, the cavernosa, to fill with blood. Hydraulic pressure causes the penis to lengthen and stiffen, now ready for sex. Every step of the process is potentially affected by the FSL. So you have to ask the question: is sex important to me?

A general rule: anything that can hurt your heart can hurt your penis, too. Just as the high blood pressure and elevated cholesterol wound arteries in the heart, the blood vessels of the penis are injured, too. The penile arteries only have a diameter of one to two millimeters compared to four millimeters in the coronary arteries. Atherosclerotic damage, endothelial injury, and cholesterol plaques compromise blood in the penis more quickly than they do in the heart. Less blood flow spells erectile dysfunction (ED), a penis not stiff enough for sex. A man will show up on his doctor's doorstep for a Viagra script but ignore chest pains for weeks. Coronary artery disease (CAD) and erectile dysfunction are so closely linked, doctors have been advised to check for CAD when a man complains of ED.

Diabetes devastates erectile capacity in several ways involving autonomic control and structure. First, it disturbs the signaling nerves to the penis and instructions are lost. No signal, no erection. Arterial insufficiency was noted in about 70% of impotent diabetics. No blood, no erection. The kicker is fibrosis of the actual erectile tissue. Picture a miracle sponge. When dry, it is about 1/8 inch thick. Dunk it in water, it blossoms to full size. The core of the penis is that sponge. With blood it blossoms. Under the microscope, ultrastructure changes in the penile tissue of diabetics are readily apparent. Elasticity and compliance are lost. The capacity of the sponge has vanished, and no erection can occur. There are medical conditions with opportunities to reverse course and recover completely, but diabetic impotence is not one of them. Without intervention, sexual dysfunction lies about ten years down the road from the diagnosis of diabetes.

Sometimes, the risk appears too far down the road to be of any immediate concern. Fortunately, erectile dysfunction only happens to older men. Right? Not at all. While it is more common with aging, young men can have problems, too. Researchers questioned a large group of soldiers, eighteen to twenty-seven years old, and found a small percentage with ED. In this group, nearly 80% were overweight or obese. In this same study, they noted that losing weight and increasing activity restored sexual function. Prevention, primarily abandoning the FSL, is the only mechanism to keep the wood.

Along with providing erection protection, dumping the FSL maintains your fertility and preserves the option to create a family. The natural sag of the testicles is necessary for sperm development. The little swimmers do not like heat and require an environment slightly cooler than 98.6 degrees. Scrotal heating, (ouch!) has been proposed as a contraceptive mechanism. A clothed man walking about has a healthy scrotal temperature of 93.2 degrees, sufficiently cool for sperm maturation and storage. When seated with thighs together, this bumps to a too-hot 96.8 degrees. Sitting on eggs is great for hatching chicks but not for developing sperm. Big legs and thighs keep the testicles insulated, equivalent to being tucked close to the body, and, again, fertility is impaired. Low sperm counts in obese men are more than just heat. The hormonal changes—less testosterone—more estrogen, affects spermatogenesis, too. The short story is that obese men are more likely to be functionally infertile, making some sperm but not of sufficient quality or quantity to create a pregnancy. In one study of over five hundred men, the ejaculate of lean men contained twenty times more sperm than that of obese men. Diabetes is a fertility disaster. Not only is erectile dysfunction more common, but ejaculation is impaired, too. Nerves in the penis, the operational switchmen allowing either sperm or urine to flow from the urethra, fail. The sperm end up in the bladder, medically termed a "retrograde" ejaculation. This is not sexually satisfying or the correct placement for pregnancy. Can it get any worse?

Excuse me, sir. Have you lost your penis? The skin in the groin is very mobile and can hold a mound of subcutaneous fat. In contrast, the penis is firmly anchored by suspensory ligaments to the pubic bone. When the suprapubic fat distends, the penis is effectively drawn into the mound. Over the course of time, a penis can shorten by inches and, in the worst case scenario, disappear completely. The medical term is "hidden penis."

With the FSL, progressive feminization is obvious, predictable, and inevitable. Testosterone gives us three important Fs: fitness, fertility, and function (sexual). The FSL shrinks the capacity to produce testosterone and begins the migration back to female.

Finally some good news and the balls of the rest of this book: Unlike ovaries, testicles remain responsive lifelong. They never fail completely; they simply slow, waiting for the right combination of signals to speed up the factory. For men, it is never too late to change.

CHAPTER 4

Floor Mats

—————

My mother's father grew up trim in the Depression but became a big-bellied man as he aged. The high school track record he set in the mile stood for almost thirty years. A picture of Grandpa in his navy uniform just after basic training shows he kept much of that form until his twenties. I remember he liked to eat, and I wonder if this was some compensation for the lean years in the 1930s. The breakfasts my grandmother would serve always included a platter of fried eggs and plenty of bacon. His exercise was swinging a splitting maul, driving a tractor, and riding horses. At Saddle Club picnics, he was proud of his appetite and never rationed the desserts. The heart attack he suffered at age fifty took years off his life and added pills to his diet. I do not know if he understood the relationship of these choices to heart disease. He was educated, but we know infinitely more about the FSL than we did forty years ago. My grandpa was forty-six when I was born, the same age I was when my daughter was born. He died when I was twenty-two, far too young. That is one reason that keeps me fit but not a fitting reason for how I got here.

Why change at all? As a doctor, I rely on the capability of individuals to make informed decisions. If you are happy with your man shape and understand the consequences of the FSL, then close this book and head to the refrigerator. This is the path of least resistance. Why change paths? Why make this investment to become something different?

Nothing comes without a cost, and there are substantial costs to losing weight and becoming fit. Maybe the time commitment is just too much. Perhaps you simply do not enjoy working out. Cutting back and eating healthy is another issue, too. If you decide against change, you are in ample company. The FSL is the path selected by the majority of men in the United States. Educated men choose to ignore the health concerns and man concerns of the FSL every day.

Starting a fitness program is like buying a car. Today, you have walked onto my lot. The goal is to ensure you drive home a new one. With any purchase, there is always a bottom line. The price of a car never goes to zero even if there are a thousand left on the lot. Rejecting the FSL mandates an informed decision followed by action. That is the bottom line. From Chapters 2 and 3, you understand the costs of your old "car" and the advantages of a new one. Intellectually, it makes sense, and you may be very nearly ready to make the deal. My job is pretty easy as you have already demonstrated your commitment in reading this book to Chapter 4. There are no dazzling Ferraris here. You will not get lowballed with a ten-minutes-a-day fitness plan. The promise is an effective, efficient program at a fair price. This offer is an investment that will pay dividends for the rest of your life. Time to close the deal.

In medical school, I was taught the Transtheoretical Model to help understand and motivate patients to make behavioral changes. This model has been criticized but, at the very least, it gives a framework to consider how people change. The model proposes individuals move from a pre-contemplation stage, where they have no particular intent to take action, to contemplation, where action is now considered. Following contemplation are preparation, action, maintenance, and, finally, termination. In my life, I have fallen away from fitness four separate times. For each fall, a different reason brought me back from the brink. There was no careful consideration, analysis of all my options, or detailed planning. I found my running shoes, started jogging, then kept with it. For men and fitness, there is only preparation, action, and maintenance.

Buy new shorts. Hit the gym. Keep with it. It sounds simple enough. Knowing full well the destination of the FSL, what keeps most men from just getting started on this new path? The answer again is simple: we are humans and remain intellectually, emotionally, and socially biased against any type of change. We develop a mindset that becomes so ingrained we continue to accept our current behavior and flounder hopelessly comfortable with our own habits. While we tend to act in our own best interests, these are more often near-term, proximate interests. Support for these concerns diminishes the thrust we feel for change. Support for the status quo comes in the form of acceptance, inertia, and cost. This is the triangle of submission.

The FSL is more a verb than a noun, a process not an event. Acceptance allows this process to continue without an attempt to change it. We live and work around others who have chosen the FSL. The belly is not uncommon in our close contacts and may be quite familiar. There is some evidence to support the person-to-person spread of obesity through subtle, unconscious influences. If you have a close friend who becomes obese, there is about a 60% chance that you will become obese, too. Our own appearance is presented in the best possible light. Weight gain may be measured from what we weighed last year, not what we weighed in college. A glance in the mirror would be telling but quickly discounted. "I'm still pretty fit. Yes, I could stand to lose a few pounds, but who couldn't? A couple of weeks of running and I would be back in shape." Daily, we measure ourselves against the world around us. "Look at him. Now that guy is fat." And we end our self-assessment with "Compared to him, I'm doing pretty well."

Submission is buttressed by inertia, active resistance to change the current state. Inertia exists in every aspect of our lives, even the things we may want to change. We settle into our homes, marriages, families, and careers. We acquire eating, drinking, sleeping, and inactivity patterns. I have to be at work by 8:00 a.m. The kids need to be picked up from soccer. We eat dinner at 6:00 p.m. I do yard work on Saturday, then church and groceries on Sunday. Intellectually, we may understand the importance of a healthy weight and adequate exercise, but to achieve that would require changing everything else, so we don't.

The cost of change is more than a gym membership, shoes, and shorts. There is the obvious cost in terms of time. Hours spent at the gym are hours away from the family, sleep, and chores. With finite hours in the day, "I have no time" is the most common argument I hear from my patients in clinic. Change also requires an admission of our current state and the apparent appraisal by the gym staff. There is the sting of self-consciousness, the awkwardness of a gym newbie, and the subtle acknowledgement of our lapse as we are passed by faster runners on the trail. Even while admitting the benefit, we may still perceive the cost of change to be too expensive.

Picture yourself attached to an elite military unit for a window of time. Looking around, you see a bunch of tough-looking guys. Strength is a requirement of the job, and a perfect score on the fitness test is expected. They get up before the sun and do physical training until breakfast. Then work begins. No bellies here. With these men as your peers, you would likely make a quick effort to get back into shape. Knowing the military, you would get plenty of mentoring and encouragement along the way. Normative influences work for positive changes, too. Within a small group, peer comparisons are a strong motivator. You get pulled into the current and are then swept along with it. The decision here is not a sudden and complete recognition of the long-term health consequences of obesity. It is alignment with the behavioral expectations of the unit. Discrepancy is the catalyst for change.

Snap back to real life where the morning begins with a doughnut. In your home or office, there is no pressure here to get fit. In fact, it may be actively discouraged with comments like, "Going to the gym again?" and "You look fine." You are used to seeing bellies around, and it is unfortunately not uncomfortable when yours starts to appear. The discrepancy has vanished, and you meld with the crowd, joining the ranks of the mediocre. Any critical reflection is avoided, and in time, your belly feels perfectly normal. If "normal" means growing boobs and losing my dick, I don't want to be normal. You have to find your discrepancy.

Doctors are taught to identify and develop the discrepancy to help facilitate behavior changes. People quit smoking in fair percentages just because a doctor asks about it. By asking, physicians set into motion cognitive dissonance and identify how a belief ("Smoking is bad for my health") and a behavior ("I still smoke") are in conflict. This discrepancy can be addressed or ignored. At times patients will soothe their discomfort with "I have cut way back." To the question "Are you planning on quitting?" my job as health coach is to help patients move from "Yes, but…" to just "Yes." Simply recognizing the discrepancy does not cause change; it only lowers the threshold to make a change. A decision still has to be made, and action has to be taken. Sometimes, the decision is easy.

In 1987, I reported to Fort Rucker, Alabama, to learn to fly helicopters for the Army Reserves. The school was nearly ten months long and busy. The Army Physical Fitness Test consists of pushups, followed by sit-ups, and then a timed two-mile run. I stayed in good shape because I had to pass this test at every stage. After graduation, I returned home with my aviator wings, the army returned to part-time status, and I promptly returned to my desk and old habits. The fitness program lapsed, and my weight crept back up. The army, whether you are active duty or reserves, requires aviators to pass a flight physical every year. Only one year out of training, I failed my flight physical. The flight surgeon told me curtly, "Your cholesterol is too high." He compared my current weight to the previous physical. In a year, I had gained almost twenty-five pounds. Again! That same damn twenty-five pounds I gained in college. That same damn twenty-five pounds I gained at my first job. I was only a little concerned about my cholesterol. I wanted to fly. Sure I wanted to eat and relax, but I wanted to fly more. The flight surgeon gave me a break: three months to bring my cholesterol down. I quickly resumed exercise and lost weight. The army got what they wanted, a healthy pilot, and I got to continue flying.

I was blessed to have an explicit decision point presented to me on a platter. You can lose weight, or you can stop flying. Rarely with the FSL is that the case. Without recognition, we slink into submission slowly, steadily. Many health issues are related to behavior, and much of what I do as a physician is health coaching. In a study of nurses involved in weight loss counseling, fat nurses were perceived as poor role models while slim nurses were perceived as having poor empathy. Credible is more important than perfect in coaching. I will never be a fitness model, but I am not embarrassed to take off my shirt at the pool. I have decent arms, but I am more proud of my cholesterol numbers. In teaching, my patients hear about my failures, struggles, and successes. This strategy was actively demonstrated by my gymnastics coach in high school.

Coach was a former gymnast himself and would demonstrate certain moves but describe others. He walked that fine line and was good enough but not too good. That made him human and real. Individually, he assessed our experience and strengths, then developed a specific program. He always had a tool or technique to goad me to the next level. He started slow and set interim goals. Through his living example, we understood the goals he set were attainable. This is an essential element for adult learners.

Men can understand fully the health concerns and the man concerns of the FSL, but these dangers seem so distant. The FSL is muddled into our lives and, most often, the discrepancy has to be presented. For my patients, I point out the impending crisis. Submission to the FSL can be tracked with the medical chart. With a "click," my patients have a graph of their weight progression. I then relate weight to blood pressure and fasting blood sugar. Once patients have the reason and relevance, they may consider action. *Dad had diabetes and had to use insulin. Dad was overweight, and I'm gaining weight. The doctor says I'm a borderline diabetic. I better do something now.* Patients do not disagree with the core issue. However, the extrinsic motivation I provide cannot compare with their intrinsic motivations that include not only health but family, career, and one hundred other distractions. The coach has little influence on athletes who are not already part of the team.

Everyone wants to change for the better. None of my patients enjoys the effect of their illness. There may not be a clear path to the solution, however. The goal may be too far down range. If the process is too involved, patients may stop even before they have started. That happened to me with flight school. The requirements were pretty simple: take a written test and pass a physical. The test was only offered on certain days. The physical required two afternoons off work and a dilated eye exam. Easy enough, but I put off my application for more than a year. My investment was about ten hours of time and, for twelve months, that seemed too expensive. An orientation ride in a Bell 47 helicopter made it seem like a bargain. What changed? I discovered something I wanted more. Decisions can be like delivering babies. Once the head is through, the rest of the baby simply follows. Once your head is committed to change, the rest will follow.

The catalyst for change can be something dramatic. At the hospital, I never let a crisis pass without comment. This is an opportunity to effect a significant change. *When did you quit smoking? Right after my heart attack.* More often than not, the catalyst is something less and may not be directly related to the behavior. *I don't want to take pills. I'd like to take my shirt off at the beach. I want to be around for my daughter's graduation. I want to run a ten K.* In retrospect, my own reasons for change were a combination of embarrassment, peer pressure, and fear. Regardless of the reason you decide to change, you still get the health benefits. In your own way, you have to discover and develop the discrepancy.

The formula for change is much like a chemical reaction. There are elements on one side of the equation with potential to react. A catalyst will allow the reaction to proceed with lower activation energy. However small, we still need that activation energy. It is that final push, the last straw, the missing piece. Add that and the change occurs. A man who shows up at a car dealer with Internet pricing, checkbook, and trade title in hand is prepared to buy a car. The elements are in place. The only item to negotiate is price. In reality, there is minimal flexibility in car pricing. The buyer has already committed to spend about 98% of the price of the car. To commit to a purchase, the salesman can reiterate the benefits, but the buyer has to believe he is getting the right deal. That is where the sweeteners come in. The price of the car might be forty thousand dollars, but the activation energy that allows the deal to proceed may be a one-hundred-dollar set of floor mats.

I'm a doctor because of floor mats. After I returned from Desert Storm, I wanted to go back to college. I had thought about getting a teaching certificate and following in my grandfather's footsteps. I had picked up enrollment materials, but I just could not make the leap. What finally got me there? A lie. Several of my friends knew my dream of returning to school. I ran into one that I had not seen for more than a year at a local hardware store. He asked me a simple question, "How is school?" I responded that I was not taking classes yet. He then asked, "When are you starting?" Without hesitation, I said, "This August." Now, I guess this was not a lie because I did start school in August. And two years later, I did not have a teaching certificate but, instead, I was headed to medical school. I had the dream, the desire, the motivation, but I was stuck. The final push, the activation energy, was simply the shame of lying—my floor mats.

Develop your discrepancy, then find your floor mats. This is as touchy-feely as this book gets.

CHAPTER 5

The Measure of a Man

———

One of my friends reviewed the first few chapters of this book and remarked it was harsh. Accurate, but harsh. I recognized this fully but declined to change a word, and he agreed. It needs to be harsh, like marine corps boot camp. In the first few days, drill instructors weed out the disinterested and unmotivated. Those remaining can be crafted into marines. Reading about testosterone, you should feel a cringe in your testicles and your brain urging action. In our times, manhood is not a gift, it is unendingly earned. Either you want it or you don't. Boot camp is not an online course and neither is the Man Plan. You do not join the brotherhood and gain the title Marine, or Man for that matter, without some slogging. The balance of the story is about your action plan, and within each chapter there is a hard lesson to apply.

Boot camp was just twelve weeks long when I went through in 1979. I was seventeen, mentally determined and physically tough; I thought of quitting every day. The drill instructors of Platoon 1039 pushed the limits and stopped just shy of my failure. All along, I knew it was an event, just twelve weeks long. In contrast, the Man Plan is for the rest of your life. The process of maintaining (or regaining) your manhood is the event. I am not your drill instructor, however. I am more the Minister of Health, delivering the motivational message and the mechanism. You must supply the sweat equity. Fortunately, we only have about one hundred years to reverse.

By geologic measures, the FSL is a recent phenomenon. In review of fossilized remains, it is fairly impossible to gain the complete picture of premodern man. The remains are too few, and the bones unearthed generally form incomplete skeletons. Average height could be largely miscalculated depending on the particular bits discovered. If the fragments and fossils found from the Neanderthal period were a "Mini-Me" equivalent, stature estimates would be wildly skewed. It does appear our more distant relatives had thicker bones and more muscular development. The relatively recent tradition of burial has provided considerable historical information regarding build. From excavations of seventeenth century graves in England, the average man's height was measured at just under sixty-six inches. Height has underlying genetic basis that is soundly influenced by the environment, chiefly nutrition. American colonists were two inches taller than their English brothers, based on evidence gathered from colonial graves. This is largely attributed to a better, more varied diet in the New World. Researchers established even the lower class was fairly well fed in the colonies.

Vertical growth occurs more or less continuously through childhood with a final acceleration during puberty. Adult height is obtained by about age eighteen in young men. In both sexes, estrogen signals closure of the epiphyseal growth plates, and little linear skeletal growth occurs beyond this point. One of the sources of historical anthropometric measurements is from the military; recruits were routinely examined on accession into service. From the Revolutionary War to World War II, a soldier's average height remained stable, about sixty-eight inches with a minor dip after the Civil War. This was partly due to the disruption of the nation's food supply. While adult height is a combination of many factors, it provides a fixed physical marker of nutritional adequacy during youth. The twentieth century introduction of mechanized farming made men nutritional lottery winners, essentially awash in food. It appears we have reached, or nearly so, our genetically programmed maximum height. The average American male now stands just over sixty-nine inches tall.

Weight is also a reflection of nutritional adequacy. Unlike height, it has capacity to increase over a man's entire life. Adult weight represents a physical balance sheet with caloric intake in one column and activity in the other. A positive balance sheet trends toward obesity. Men clearly have the capacity to grow. At his death in 1809, Daniel Lambert, billed as "The fattest man in Britain," tipped the scales at 739 pounds. Historically, a stout man was considered financially prosperous and healthy to boot. As early as 1770, organizations began offering life insurance in the colonies. Actuaries evaluated policy applicants and sought to minimize risk in issuing life insurance contracts. Thin applicants were routinely rejected as some degree of chubbiness was valued as a buffer against disease. During this period, pneumonia and tuberculosis were among the leading causes of death. Underweight men were more likely to succumb to these pulmonary infections.

Shortly after its invention in 1885, the penny scale appeared as a street corner novelty in America. Men could now weigh themselves, and it prompted the obvious question, "What should I weigh?" Life insurance companies provided an answer in the form of standard height and weight charts based on information gathered from their applicants. In 1900, a thirty-year-old man standing sixty-eight inches tall weighed, on average, 154 pounds. This figure may be somewhat overstated as it required some financial soundness to consider purchasing life insurance. The underprivileged may have been lighter but not represented. Based on trends over the past forty years, we are still swelling to our genetic maximum weight. By 1960, average weight for men aged twenty to seventy-four had crept to 166 pounds. When measured again in 2002, the average weight for this group jumped to 191 pounds, reflecting another 15% bump in just forty-two years. The world's fattest man now approaches 1,400 pounds, nearly doubling Daniel Lambert's record.

Weight remains the most common measurement men use to assess their health status. An issue I had when I first returned to the gym in 2004 was my rate of change; it appeared to be zero. Though I was working out almost every day, the scale did not budge. It was horribly demoralizing and, like boot camp, I felt like quitting. Only my pending deployment to Iraq kept me with the program. When I finally started tuning down my calorie intake and ramping up weightlifting, the pounds started coming off. Without a doubt, even when I first started working out, there were subtle changes taking place. On a day-to-day basis, it was imperceptible, akin to emptying a bathtub with a tablespoon. I was anchored on weight, relying on the one tool I had at home, my scale. Daily weights can vary by more than a few pounds depending on hydration status, meal timing, and last bathroom break. There is still a scale in my home, and I use it several times a week, always in the morning, standing in shorts with an empty bladder. This gives another bit of information to help tweak my diet and workout program. Unfortunately, weight alone is fairly meaningless without some specifics. Two hundred and fifty pounds can be bodybuilder fit or morbidly obese.

Body mass index (BMI) is commonly referenced in medical literature. A Belgian mathematician, Adolphe Quetelet, developed it nearly two hundred years ago in his study of human physical characteristics as a method for classifying sedentary individuals with average body structure. The index was formulated for population studies, what Quetelet called "Social Physics." The formula is straightforward: body weight divided by the square of height; many online BMI calculators are available. For years it was called the Quetelet Index until the term Body Mass Index was coined in 1972.

$$\frac{\text{Mass (kgs)}}{(\text{Height (meters)})^2}$$

BMI places men into descriptive categories ranging from Underweight to Morbidly Obese. In medical studies, patients are grouped by BMI to assess morbidity and mortality trends. Though it is entirely unsuitable for individuals, BMI unfortunately remains widely used by doctors and trainers to document and discuss obesity. Beyond unsuitable, it is shamefully inaccurate for this purpose. BMI makes no precise assumption about body composition. In a par-

BMI Categories	
Underweight	16.5 – 18.4
Normal	18.5 – 24.9
Overweight	25 – 29.9
Obese	30+
Morbidly Obese	40+

ticular study, BMI identified obesity in 19.1% of the population. The true figure was closer to 44% when actual body fat was measured. My BMI is just under 25; by close inspection, no one would say I am overweight. Arnold Schwarzenegger was 74 inches tall and weighed about 250 pounds when he was competing for Mr. Universe. His calculated BMI was 32.1. Obese? The bottom line is: understand the application of BMI when reading medical studies, but do not use it to assess your health or track your progress.

On an atomic level, the top five elements in the human body are oxygen, nitrogen, hydrogen, carbon, and calcium. While the body contains about fifty of nature's elements, these five account for 98% of man's body weight. On a molecular level, a prototypical seventy-kilogram man is about 60% water. The balance is lipids (19%), proteins (15%), and minerals (5%), loosely representing fat, muscle, and bone, respectively. These compartments have the capacity to change and can be changed. Water, on the other hand, just tags along for the ride, moving proportionally with the other components. For our purposes, we can partition a man into just two compartments: Fat and Fat Free Mass (FFM). Fat is self-explanatory. FFM is everything else: muscle, bone,

$$FFM = Total\ Body\ Weight - Fat$$

water, and the small fraction of giblets that are none of the above.

If you are just measuring with a scale, a ten-pound weight drop seems like an unqualified success but, in reality, it may be a mixed blessing. Caloric restriction is an economic crisis of sorts in the body. The brain, liver, kidneys, and heart always have to be fed at the expense of every other body system. When consumed calories are reduced below basal metabolic requirements, the body looks to both stored fat and skeletal muscle as sources of energy. In usual weight loss (basic caloric restriction), about 70% of the reduction is attributed to metabolized fat. If you are just measuring with a scale, you may gain a false sense of security from your weight. A friend of mine and I are exactly the same height and nearly the same weight. We both pass army weight standards easily. His measured body fat is 28%, mine is closer to 12%. Our waists differ by six inches. His build is an example of normal weight obesity, too much fat (visceral) and, perhaps, not enough muscle.

The essence of the Man Plan is losing fat, building muscle, and strengthening bones. How do we assess the effectiveness of our program? The answer is body composition via tracking fat and FFM. When you begin the program, you will want both baseline weight and body composition. Body weight is easy to measure with your home scale. Body fat is another story. Given that 100% accuracy requires burning a body to ash, I am willing to accept an estimate.

The army uses a conservative height/weight chart for recruits. If you fall above the range for your height, body fat is measured by taping. Only two circumferential measurements, the neck and abdomen, are required. The neck is measured just below the Adam's apple. The abdomen is measured at the belly button. These two numbers along with age, height, and weight are plugged into an impossibly complex formula to produce a body fat estimate. The formula makes certain assumptions about typical body fat distribution. Inaccuracy is introduced because genetics play a sizeable role in determining where fat accumulates, subcutaneous or visceral. Though the tape measure is a simple instrument, as you can expect, the taping process is subject to some interindividual variations in measurement techniques. Army applicants rejected for having too much body fat can be retaped at some point to try again. In reviewing entrance physicals, I have seen neck sizes increase by an inch and bellies drop by four inches over the course of a month without any change in weight. Hmm. The formula is available online and, with some assistance (and honesty) in taping, reproducible. Men tend to lose abdominal-visceral fat first, so the army method can validate early progress in your program.

Skin fold thickness is also used to estimate body fat. The skin over certain muscle groups in the chest, abdomen, back, arms, and thighs is pinched with special calipers. Measurements are taken at three to eight points depending on the particular method. The total thickness is compared to height to estimate body fat. In theory, the measured subcutaneous fat is representative of total body fat. In actuality, this may not be true for an individual. The measurements rely on the caliper operator being accurate and consistent in both placement and pinch of the caliper. Some calipers are designed to give a consistent pinch, leaving only placement as a source of error. As with taping, the formulas used for skin calipers make certain assumptions including where body fat is located. Individuals with a higher percentage of visceral fat will give a lower body fat reading. As with taping, a trained helper is necessary to take these measurements. It is fairly accurate and reproducible, and the only cost is for the calipers.

One technique that requires no human measurement is bioelectrical impedance analysis (BIA). Muscles and bone have high water content and are good conductors. Fat, on the other hand, is a poor conductor. BIA sends a small electric current through the body and measures resistance, the proxy for fat. Typical BIA devices are gripped with both hands, with the current passing through your arms and chest. Newer fitness scales may have a built-in BIA capacity, using your bare feet as the contact points. The usual BIA monitor requires age, height, weight, and gender inputs to estimate body fat percentage. Others make adjustments for physical activity and have an "athlete" setting. There are some cautions regarding BIA estimates as they can be affected by hydration status. For example, measuring after a meal or working out may significantly affect your results. I purchased a simple model and use it at a recommended time: after waking but before showering, eating, or drinking. I like BIA as the operator error is nil and, with controls for hydration status, the results are consistent and reproducible.

The gold standard for body fat measurement remains hydrodensitometry, the medical term, I suppose, for "dunking in water." Fat, muscle, and bone have different densities. Muscle sinks and fat floats. Weight on dry land is compared to weight in water and, again, through a complex formula that involves estimating lung volumes, a body fat measurement is produced. The ceremonial dunking needs to be completed several times with the results averaged. In the literature, I have seen it described as "cumbersome and uncomfortable" in addition to "limited availability and expensive."

There are also specialized pods that measure body volume to approximate composition. Even this technique is subject to some estimation because of the retained air in the lungs after a complete exhalation. Imaging techniques including dual energy X-ray absorptiometry (DEXA), Magnetic Resonance Imaging (MRI), and Computed Tomography (CT) have been used to estimate body fat. These are typically reserved for medical studies and generally unavailable to the common man. Where available, they are fairly expensive.

I am not convinced that any of the advanced techniques are a good value. Taping, calipers, and BIA can be completed at home on your schedule. Daily, weekly, monthly. While they are not 100% accurate, they are internally consistent if you are externally consistent in their application. The initial investment might be $1.47 for a cloth tape measure or $30 for a handheld BAI monitor. In contrast, DEXA may cost $100 for each measurement. If you still think you need a DEXA scan, note there is good agreement between BIA measures and DEXA scans. My advice is to choose one basic technique and stick with it; the results between BIA, taping, and calipers are not interchangeable. Regardless of the method you choose, remember, it is only a marker and a way of keeping score.

Body composition is the penny scale of our century. As soon as we were able to measure it, men began asking, "What is an ideal body fat?" The army regulations state the maximum acceptable body fat percentage for a new recruit age twenty-five is 26%. The army expects to give you some physical training and health education, so after entry the percentage drops to 22%. From my perspective, 22% body fat is a D grade, passing but clearly not ideal. It is unacceptably close to 25% body fat, where the risk of metabolic syndrome and other health issues climb. On the other end of the spectrum, experts opine that 5% is the minimal essential body fat for a man. The American Council on Exercise notes that athletes range from 6-13% body fat, fit individuals have 14-17%, and an average man is 18-24%. Regardless of weight, more than 25% body fat in a man is considered obese.

Body Fat	
5%	Minimal
6-13%	Athletic
14-17%	Fit
18-24%	Average
>25%	Obese

It seems the body fat-health risk curve is U-shaped. Too little body fat is just as bad as too much for entirely different reasons. I would venture that 10% body fat is a functional minimum for most men. This is based on studies of measured body fat across a spectrum of sports from rugby to running. In 1943, the Metropolitan Life Insurance Company produced standard height-weight tables. Through subsequent revisions they have become known as "ideal" weight charts. The tables simply reflect the range of weights for men who have the lowest overall mortality. They account for frame size (small, medium, large) but not body fat or composition. For a medium-framed man of average height (sixty-nine inches) the "ideal" weight ranges from 146 to 158 pounds. I did some rough calculations and guessed that 12% body fat was at the low end of the Metropolitan Life scale. Using this as a starting point, I calculated body fat at the upper end to be 18%. This favorably compares to the American Council of Exercise's categories of Athletic and Fit. I believe that 10-18% body fat is a wide, reasonable, and attainable corridor for men. Understand, however, that all body fat measurements (except burning) are estimates and vary day to day. In reality, body fat is an esoteric figure. A fitness program is about change. Body fat measurement is a tool that only describes the direction and magnitude of change, not a precise number. Rather than celebrating a particular nadir of 14.04% body fat, I monitor my body fat trend over a month's time as I adjust my Man Plan.

Ten percent body fat is something I have never been able to obtain despite my grand understanding of exercise physiology. In athletes, the ideal body composition is an intersection of speed, agility, and power required for the sport. For men, ideal body composition is unique to the owner, a reflection of priorities and competing demands, a human collision between aspirations and reality. It is not a static goal but moves with age, jobs, relationships, seasons, and one hundred other factors. In writing a book, I did not have the opportunity to devote 100% of my time and complete the project in two months. My intersection of work, spouse, daughter, and sleep left me just thirty minutes a day to write. These limits gave me focus, urgency, and efficiency. My gym time is limited by those same commitments to about sixty minutes a day. When I train, I have the same focus, urgency, and efficiency. Research lead to the choice, tempo, and even intensity of my exercise program. Gym time is synergized by actions during the remaining twenty-three hours of the day. In every sense, I have become the living demonstration of the Man Plan and still a work in progress. Through the balance of this book, I will share these tried and true strategies as you read and contemplate your own ideal body.

When I returned from Desert Storm in 1991, I had a slight itch to go back to school for an advanced degree. A US Army Reserve friend of mine entered law school after his return from Vietnam some twenty years prior. He described the process of tests, applications, and interviews. When he was accepted, he stopped working, moved, and started school. He became a successful attorney and continued part-time military service as an army aviator. In hearing his story, I was stirred but also staggered by the requisite sacrifice. Essentially he said, "All you have to change is everything." My itch faded and I set that dream on a shelf for a while. Years later, after I had finished medical school, others asked me about my journey. Though I tested, applied, interviewed, sold, moved, borrowed, started, struggled, and finished, it was nothing about sacrifice. It was all about choice. I chose to pursue medicine as a career and have reaped the benefits professionally and personally ever since.

Hard Lesson #1: The Man Plan is not about sacrifice. It is about choice. Fitness and health are no accident. Application of the Man Plan is a conscious decision followed by continuous effort operating against current societal, environmental, and genetic pressures. In time, it will not seem hard, just part of the plan.

Homework Assignment #1—Start Keeping Score
Measure your weight and body fat, then calculate your FFM. Record all of this in your log book. (Did I forget to mention you need a log book?)

CHAPTER 6

Engaging Autopilot

———

By definition, diet is the sum of the food consumed by an individual. It has become synonymous with caloric restriction and weight loss. For me, this descriptive term conjures up some distasteful childhood memories. Periodically, my mother would embark on a peculiar weight loss program. She baked a fillet of turbot fish along with several slices of squash sprinkled with cinnamon. She ate this consistently for lunch and dinner. From my recollection, it did not rise to the level of bland as that would imply it had some flavor. After a few weeks and several lost pounds, the baking would stop and the pungent odor of scorched fish would slowly fade from the kitchen. I now understand her food choices were good: high protein, low calorie, and low fat. But her method of weight loss was fundamentally incorrect. She went on a diet like going on vacation: a brief event lasting a few weeks and a few pounds. The actual process is more like rambling down the Appalachian Trail.

Short and simple: body weight is a balance sheet. More calories consumed than expended equals weight gain. More calories expended than consumed equals weight loss. This is a universal truth. Nearly every day I have a patient complain, "I just cannot lose weight," and some continue with, "I only eat once a day. Others declare, "I never eat." This explanation is either a gross exaggeration or a miracle of thermodynamics I should document and publish. I do concede there are a few medical disorders that cause men to put on pounds. Progressive weight gain is the most common symptom of Cushing's syndrome, a rare condition, where excess cortisol drives appetite and produces a distinctive pattern of fat deposition. Hypothyroidism slows metabolism making it much easier to gain and maintain excess weight. Any number of drugs from antidepressants to anticonvulsants may cause some weight gain. These particular medical issues are fairly easy to sort out with a bit of due diligence by a physician. The remaining 99.99% of us either eat too much, exercise too little, or both.

Weight loss becomes an entirely predictable outcome when we increase activity, reduce intake, and create a negative balance sheet. In controlled situations, we can rather accurately predict how much weight will be lost. Thank God for US Army Rangers. Not only do they defend the country in a most aggressive style, they allow themselves to be studied while they earn the coveted ranger tab. The candidates are put through an extremely rigorous eight-week course under simulated combat conditions in mountain, swamp, and desert environments. They move constantly, training twenty hours per day. Stress is high; food and sleep are in short supply. Activity is mandated and intake is strictly limited. Each troop gets on average 2,800 calories per day. A decent amount of food until you consider they are burning nearly 4,000 calories every day. Running the numbers, a 1,200-calorie-a-day deficit for sixty days is 72,000 calories total, a debt equivalent to twenty pounds of fat. In eight weeks, the typical ranger course trainee will lose 12% of their body weight and burn off fully half of their body fat. The numbers work.

Ranger candidates are hard-core motivated troops, their food is rationed, and they are literally under the gun to keep moving. Arriving at ranger training, soldiers already have a high level of fitness and at the completion emerge very, very lean. It puts into perspective the substantial effort it takes to quickly lose twenty pounds. When we loosen the controls some and simply stipulate increased activity, the results are pretty good, too.

US Army recruits differ in their stature and stamina when they swear into the military. The transition from civilian to soldier begins with Basic Combat Training (BCT). In this ten-week course, individuals learn the fundamentals of military life and essential army skills. Throughout the process, there is a variety of physical training daily from intense calisthenics to recreational games. There are no restrictions in the chow hall but expressly limited snacking opportunities. BCT engages recruits in about nine hours of activity per day, shifting their usual focus from knowledge-based work and sedentary activities to motion. At the end of training, seventy days more or less, soldiers emerge with 11% less body fat and more lean muscle mass.

It is crystal clear in these two structured environments that men can lose weight. With the possible exception of police and fire academies, there are virtually no civilian equivalents to boot camp or ranger training. What if we loosen the controls even further and shrink training intensity? Consider a program where men are coached to exercise and are allowed, in fact, encouraged, to keep the same caloric intake. Even still, they lose fat and put on muscle. It does take longer, as expected, and the changes occur over months not weeks. In one study that required jogging just twenty miles a week, men lost an average of eleven pounds of fat and gained three pounds of muscle in eight months. In the same study, a different group was only required to jog twelve miles a week. Their results were still significant but proportionately less than the twenty-mile per week group. The study conclusion agrees with the laws of thermodynamics: weight loss is all about caloric insufficiency whether created by increasing expenditures, decreasing intake, or both. Weight loss math works not just for rangers and recruits but ordinary men, too.

Whether you are a soldier, athlete, or ordinary man, your body is a reflection of the demands placed on it. In the move from labor to knowledge-based work and sedentary play, energy demands decreased. As the average man's life changed from working his back and biceps to using his brain, we have made downward adjustments in daily caloric intake. By and large, individual calorie consumption fairly well matches individual energy expenditures. Human appetite regulation is a decent, but not perfect, system. As I noted in Chapter 2, we generally only have a twenty-calorie mismatch per day. This, however, translates into twenty pounds over ten years. With changes in stress and sleep related to careers, family, marriage, or divorce, we can add weight much more quickly—in my case, over twenty-five pounds in just under a year. Because the appetite is always driving to maintain weight, it is difficult to know exactly how much to eat. On the other hand, when we return to our "caveman" roots, genetically programmed behaviors emerge to guide our food choices.

Many solid studies show that activity is an appetite modulator. The relative food deprivation in ranger training led these men to eat anything they could reach. I got to observe a feeding frenzy firsthand. During flight school, part of our training was to shuttle ranger trainees during the Florida phase of their course. We learned about moving troops; they learned about air assaults. In a decades-old unspoken agreement, they were granted a free pass on board our aircraft to eat anything we gave them. For the ten-minute ride they could chow down. But nothing left the aircraft except what was in their bellies. No one refused peanut butter and jelly sandwiches from our cooler. Instinct took over and they just inhaled them. In Basic Combat Training, no drill instructors coached the army recruits what to eat, but these new soldiers intuitively matched their intake to their energy expenditure. Jogging twenty miles a week, about four hours of activity, moved the body weight set point in ordinary men. Their bodies reflected it with more muscle and less fat.

The human body is a responsive instrument, and intense training leads to a tight modulation of intake. When I have been part of organized athletics in school and the military, we trained for several hours each day; I did not worry about eating. You might believe that hard training would lead to overeating, but the truth is the opposite. Yes, I was burning enough calories to eat anything I wanted. It just happened I did not care to eat so much. What I wanted and needed was a body fit for my sport. The regular, intense activity guided me to that end. While there are some genetic boundaries, men have a large capacity to adjust to their unique athletic situation. Comparison of athletes from different sports provides a living demonstration. Throughout monitored training, elite runners and swimmers ate about the same number of calories per day. Both groups had intense workouts, and daily energy output was roughly equal to their intake. The average body fat in the runners was 7% while the swimmers averaged 12%. Extra weight in running is a tax you pay for every mile. Competitive runners responsively drop their fat to just above the minimal essential with some reserve for the distance. Fat in swimming does not carry much of a penalty. For swimmers, body fat smoothes curves, provides insulation, and increases buoyancy. With tough training, these athletes got the bodies they needed to compete. Every man's body composition represents the dynamic intersection of competing demands, not only athletic training but work, family, stress, and sleep.

Without certain demands, the process goes to hell quickly. There is no overload switch in the brain that says, "You weigh too much, eat less." In fact, merely eating less, even if you are overweight, gives you a hungry brain. Exercise is the force that "right sizes" our intake and blunts behavioral responses to stress. The more intense the training, the better the body is in tune with energy needs. The sedentary lifestyle eliminates this critical input, and we lose the ability to determine how much to eat. This is similar to flying in the clouds where visual references are lost. Without eyes on the instruments or the horizon, we get disoriented and make poor decisions. Pilots spiral into the earth; men spiral into obesity. Researchers theorize that stress increases brain activity, consuming more calories. As the brain runs solely on glucose, it "pulls" this from the bloodstream and the rest of the body. Sensing a drop in blood sugar, appetite switches on and we seek out food to calm it. This pattern can become ingrained as "comfort eating," using caloric dense foods to mitigate the brain's glucose pull. In a manner, this stabilizes energy flow to the brain but at a significant cost to the body.

Athletes may cede conscious control and rely on innate behaviors to guide the qualities and quantities of the food they eat. During vigorous training, appetite goes on autopilot. In my usual day, there is no particular three-hour stretch where I can drop by the gym to exercise. I only have one hour, at most, on the way home from work. Without the metabolic autopilot of the intensely training athlete, men have to "cerebralize" the process, employing both resolve and restraint. Mild and moderate exercise give us stability control, but deliberate inputs are absolutely necessary.

A man requires a certain amount of energy for normal body functions. The brain, heart, liver, and kidneys always need to be fed. An average sedentary man burns roughly

20% of his calories in activity; the other 80% goes toward the essential processes, including generating body heat. Basal metabolic rate (BMR) is the theoretical amount of energy required for basic life functions while an individual is at rest, the 80% piece. Most trainers use BMR in some form or fashion as a tool for monitoring and adjusting caloric intake. An accurate measurement of BMR requires a twelve-hour fast so the gut is resting, too. Oxygen consumption is then measured for ten to thirty minutes while the subject is reclining quietly in a dim, warm room. Availability and cost keep direct BMR measurements out of reach but for practical purposes, only a solid estimate is necessary. Online calculators are available; these rely on age, weight, and height. When compared to directly measured BMR, they are fairly accurate because activity, and therefore the contributions of skeletal muscle, has been dropped out. BMR represents the bare-bones minimal caloric intake per day for a man doing nothing. Anything less would be accurately described as starvation. To gauge how many calories a man actually needs, BMR must be adjusted for activity, using a factor of 1.2 for sedentary men and ramping up progressively to 1.9 for intensely active men. BMR is a number to know and helps put an eating plan in perspective. Like any other cockpit indicator, it is something to monitor but should not become the focus of the process.

BMR Factors	
Sedentary	1.2
Lightly Active	1.375
Moderately Active	1.55
Very Active	1.725
Intensely Active	1.9

Low fat. Low carbohydrate. Low calorie. All of these diets will produce weight loss when expenditures exceed intake. Even the one-meal-a-day program can bring about weight loss, but the metabolic consequences offset any potential benefits. Programs that raise cholesterol and blood pressure unintentionally are patently counterproductive as well. Activity overload, equivalent to ranger training (2,800 calories in, 4,000 calories out), also produces weight loss at a significant physical cost. Over the eight-week program, men lost not only body fat but muscle mass, too, as their bodies sought the means to sustain the pace. Any program that produces muscle loss is undesirable and unsustainable. A sustainable plan must maintain or build lean muscle while reducing body fat. Army recruits and ordinary men both created sustainable plans by simply adding exercise and following their body's signals. A man has the genetic and vital capacity to respond suitably and forge the body necessary to meet a range of demands.

I had heard for many years that losing weight via caloric restriction alone (traditional dieting) would ultimately lead to increases in body fat. Physiology research demonstrates this old wives' tale about weight cycling is true. I noted earlier that dropping calories creates a hungry brain and a crisis in the body. The usual weight loss from caloric restriction is about 70% fat and 30% skeletal muscle. When the diet ends, the hungry brain and old habits resume and the weight comes back, not the same 70/30 mix but closer to 100% body fat. Muscle builds with stimulus and time; fat builds with any excess calories. The ranger trainees were stressed by continuous exertion, food deprivation, and elemental exposure. Calories were mobilized from fat and skeletal muscle, and every man lost a significant amount of weight. At the six-week mark, some men were approaching minimum essential fat, about 5%. During the final two weeks, the leanest men lost mostly skeletal muscle. Of course, starved but otherwise healthy men rebound when fed. Once training was over, the newly minted rangers resumed eating. On an ad lib diet, weight bounced back and rose even higher than entry weight by nearly twelve pounds. No big deal until you recognize this bonus weight was virtually 100% fat. For these lean rangers, body fat ballooned to 21% just three months after they pinned on their tabs.

In ordinary men, weight cycling erodes body composition much more subtly. An example is a 200-pound man who loses 10 pounds by caloric restriction. His body fat prior to the loss was 20%, just average, and he ends his diet with a new 190-pound body sporting 17.3% body fat. When he stops dieting after a month or so, the hungry brain takes over his appetite. Throughout the next year, he regains the lost weight, not the fat and muscle he lost but 10 pounds of pure fat. His weight is back to where he started, 200 pounds, but his body fat is now 21.5%. Repeat this cycle annually for the next four years. Our example man has aged five years and still weighs 200 pounds. Unfortunately, his body fat has climbed to 26%, now in the obese range. His FFM has dropped from 160 pounds to 148. Relying solely on caloric restriction to maintain weight works for very few men. The hungry brain with its years of evolutionary experience almost always wins.

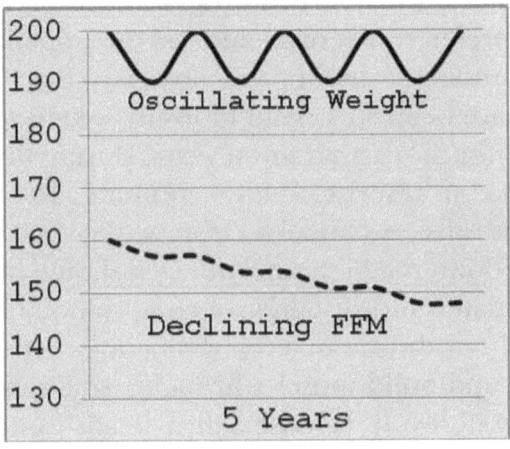

More than just losing weight, the Man Plan is about modifying body composition—building lean body mass (muscle)—while shedding fat. Calorie-restricted diets produce weight loss but flare appetite hormones and create a hungry brain that will overpower even the most prepared. Weight is ultimately regained as body fat. The key to the Man Plan is activity, eliminating "sedentary" in the FSL. Adding activity establishes a new set point, and a man's body spontaneously moves to it. Unlike women, men do not have to defend fat stores to maintain fertility, and this allows us to lose fat more easily. Rather than setting appetite on fire, as we expect, exercise modulates it, providing a reason and quantity to eat. When the calorie deficits are produced from exercise, there is no associated appetite flare. In a nutshell, exercise will burn glucose and free fatty acids from the bloodstream. Glycogen stores in the liver and muscles are tapped to replace blood glucose. The body begins lipolysis, breaking down fat, to liberate stored energy. As long as there are sufficient stores, energy spent in exercise is not replaced through increased intake. I suppose, with exercise, the body is bright enough to know when extra calories reside on the belly.

Numerous weight loss programs rely on counting calories. I prefer to exercise and let the appetite and intake adjust automatically. For the most part, this has worked for me. I have been successful in losing weight and keeping it off now for more than seven years. During this time, I have never had to resort to calorie counting. To me, that seems a bit obsessive, essentially staring at the speedometer while driving down the highway. Your eyes should be on the road. The initiator and sustainer of composition change is activity. Without drastic or even deliberate diet changes, men lose fat and build muscle through regular exercise. Learn it, know it, live it. Intense activity leads to intense tuning, but even moderate activity, jogging twenty miles per week, leads to genuine progress. Adding a bit of conscious control further enhances and maintains the process.

Prior to my deployment in 2004, I was thirty pounds overweight, the product of zero exercise and overeating. My "get fit" plan added back activity, running at first and then adding weight lifting. This strategy had worked quickly several times in the past, and I assumed it would again. After two months of my program, there was little change, at least how I was measuring it. Looking back, I was probably on the ordinary man weight loss trajectory, one and a half pounds per month. At that rate, it would take twenty months to meet my goal. I now had only four months and still thirty pounds to go. Salvation came in the form of a food diary, a little spiral notebook where I charted everything I consumed. The record quickly revealed the pattern of stress eating and a horrible underestimation of intake. Such recall bias is human nature. When people are asked to remember what they have eaten, calories are routinely underestimated by 15-30%. Food diaries add insight as well as accountability. This is the conscious control element of the Man Plan.

In a large fitness study, the predictors of weight loss were maintaining a food diary and adding activity. More activity, more weight lost. More diary entries, more weight loss. Even under the worst of conditions this plan works. During my 2009 Iraq tour, I started the Biggest Loser contest in Iraq on the forward operating base (FOB) where I was working. About fifteen overweight soldiers signed up. There were only three rules: add at least thirty minutes of exercise per day, keep a complete food diary, and weigh in every Sunday. We weighed the contestants, measured their body fat, and let the contest roll for twelve weeks. One soldier immediately realized he was drinking eight-plus sodas per day, adding more than a thousand calories to his caloric intake. Every man who followed these simple rules lost weight, about ten pounds over twelve weeks. You might say these men had some special motivation to sign up and that lead to their ultimate success. You are now finishing Chapter 6 of this book; I would suggest you have an even greater level of motivation than these combat troops. Take the next step.

Hard Lesson #2: A man's body is the dynamic intersection of demands placed on it by all forces. An athletic demand is absolutely necessary to actively engage intake controls.

Homework Assignment #2—Resume conscious control

Calculate your BMR, then determine your sedentary caloric needs (1.2 factor) and intense activity needs (1.9 factor). This is your range. Start a food diary. Record anything and everything you consume.

CHAPTER 7

Preflight

————

The morning is cold and windy with more than an hour to go before sunrise. I have already reviewed the aircraft logbook, a green binder that thoroughly details the maintenance history and status of the UH-60 Blackhawk helicopter. After stowing my gear in the cockpit, by flashlight I begin the preflight ritual, a patterned visual and physical inspection of the aircraft before launching on today's mission. Only after all the systems are inspected is the aircraft truly ready. Most, in fact nearly all, preflight inspections reveal nothing out of place or in need of repair. But we still do them. The cost-benefit ratio is very good and the twenty to thirty minutes I invest may save a multimillion dollar aircraft plus fourteen lives. Early in training I found a cracked stabilizer, and it kept me on the lookout the rest of my career. Prior to embarking on your Man Plan, you need a brief inspection, too. A preparticipation medical examination is something even six-year-old ball players get before joining a Little League team.

For high school and college athletes, there are well-researched practice guidelines available for doctors to follow. The family and personal medical histories of the student give the physician clues regarding overall health and potential concerns. After a small battery of focused questions and a head-to-toe physical examination, the physician may choose to order more testing to effectively rule in or rule out certain critical conditions. Very few in this younger age group are restricted from competing based on preparticipation exams. Despite a methodical process, we generally do not uncover anything of concern. Sudden death of a team member is a complex tragedy but also quite uncommon. Within a ten-year period, millions of high school and college athletes competed in the United States; 160 died. As these deaths were almost always related to heart conditions, specifically hypertrophic cardiomyopathy and congenital coronary artery anomalies, the core of the preparticipation examination is the cardiac evaluation. Heart conditions can be present from infancy and lie dormant until tested in practice or competition. In young athletes, doctors are looking for signs and listening for symptoms of these rare conditions that might prompt a focused cardiac workup.

For the group of men well beyond high school resuming an exercise program, the preparticipation examination should include a comprehensive assessment of the heart, too. In men over age thirty-five, fully 85% of deaths related to exercise are from coronary artery disease (CAD). This is not a warning to seek safety on the couch, rather an admonishment to meet with your physician. True, vigorous activity increases the incidence of a heart attack in men who do not work out regularly. In the United States, heart disease is the number one cause of death for men over age twenty. In men with pre-existing CAD, those susceptible to heart attacks, exercise may trigger an acute event. The other side of the coin clearly shows regular physical activity drops the overall risk of heart attack by interrupting the development of CAD. Identifying preexisting, silent CAD is one primary goal of the preparticipation examination. If you currently exercise, I would nonetheless recommend a visit with your physician. Regardless of your conditioning, cardiac screening still has a value for risk factor identification and modification. Even ultramarathoners can develop CAD.

Throughout the visit, doctors are looking for signs and listening for symptoms that might prompt more questions or testing. Development of coronary disease in men is an intersection of heredity and modifiable risk factors. A few men will have the genetic predisposition to develop heart troubles early in life. Family medical history regarding heart disease in close relatives, especially early deaths (less than age fifty) from heart conditions, provides this critical clue. In most men, however, without intervention, CAD builds slowly and progressively. The majority will show no overt symptoms for decades, others may have mild symptoms but ignore them or misinterpret their significance. A gentleman I was seeing in my clinic one afternoon complained several times of nausea, then vomited in my trash can. He apologized for showing up at my office sick. Really, he did. He thought he had indigestion, I thought he had the flu. His ashen color worried me, so I sent him directly to the ER. We both were mistaken; he was actually having a heart attack. The most common CAD prodromal symptoms are exertional chest pain, excessive dyspnea (shortness of breath), unusual fatigue, and unexplained syncope (passing out or nearly so).

Prodromal Symptoms
Exertional Chest Pain
Excessive Dyspnea
Unusual Fatigue
Unexplained Syncope

Modifiable risk factors for CAD include high cholesterol, high blood pressure, high blood sugar (and diabetes), and smoking. Of course you should know if you smoke; the other factors can be checked with a blood pressure cuff and standard blood tests. With the right combination of age, symptoms, and risk factors, additional investigation is warranted. For certain high-risk occupations, the threshold for concern is set very low. For example, in-air death of a pilot is catastrophic; high cholesterol levels in an army aviator over age forty might trigger a thorough cardiac workup. The typical screening examination, however, is a staged pro-

Modifiable Risk Factors
Smoking
High cholesterol
High blood pressure
High blood sugar

cess with successive tests giving either comfort in stopping or sufficient reason to continue with additional tests. The doctor wants to determine whether the fatigue of climbing stairs is related to heart muscle ischemia or simply being out of shape. The goal, ruling out significant heart disease, is balanced against cost, both financial and health risks, from the testing itself.

Blood tests required for a cardiac workup are fasting blood sugar and lipid panel, both completed after a full twelve-hour fast. The physical exam should include listening to your heart with a stethoscope for murmurs, perhaps while completing Valsalva's maneuver or straining. The electrocardiogram (EKG) is a simple office test, inexpensive, noninvasive, and informative. I would lay money down that any adult showing up for a preparticipation exam will get one. If your family medical history and personal medical history are bland and your exam and lab tests are reasonably normal, your workup might stop here with a blessing to resume exercising.

If there are even minor concerns, the workup might continue further to identify silent CAD. Your doctor might recommend exercise stress testing, where sequential EKGs and blood pressure readings are completed while you jog on a treadmill. The speed and incline increase at regular intervals until you are seemingly sprinting up a mountain. The heart's response to progressively increasing demand is noted, and the test typically stops when you reach the target heart rate set by your physician. In general, the longer you are able to go, the more sensitive the test is in predicting CAD. The echocardiogram, an ultrasound evaluation of the structure and function of the heart, is another noninvasive test. This can be completed at rest, after exercise, or both. Effort allows a better look at heart valve function. Just like on preflight inspections, more often than not, these tests will be normal, indicating low risk of CAD.

With strong indications of CAD, the physician may want a closer look at your coronary arteries and perfusion of the heart muscle. For myocardial perfusion studies, an injected radioactive tracer distributes in the heart muscle proportional to blood flow. The distribution is measured at rest and then after exercise; differences in flow imply clogged coronary arteries. The gold standard for evaluating coronary arteries remains cardiac catheterization and angiography. A catheter inserted in the femoral artery is guided to the heart and used to inject radiopaque dye into the various arteries of the heart. Narrowed vessels, CAD, can be visualized and quantitatively measured. They can also be treated by propping open a vessel with a tiny metal cage (stenting) if the stenosis is significant. Unfortunately, cardiac catheterization also carries a small chance of heart attack and stroke, so the value of the study must be weighed against this risk. A relatively new alternative is coronary computed tomographic angiography (CCTA). With this test, after contrast material is injected into a vein, a detailed CT scan of the heart shows arteries and also the calcium buildup that occurs with CAD. CCTA has a 99% negative predictive value. If this test does not show CAD, you almost certainly do not have it. CCTA does expose you to more than a trivial amount of radiation, increasing the risk of some cancers. Again, the small risk of the test must be considered by you and your physician against the benefit of knowing.

> **The Usual Cardiac Evaluation Sequence**
> History, Physical, Labs, EKG
> →Exercise stress testing/Echocardiography
> →Myocardial Perfusion Studies
> →Coronary Angiography/CCTA

As I have stated several times before, more often than not, men complete the cardiac workup without uncovering anything notable. Even so, a methodical workup has value, given that 50% of the time, the first concerning symptom of CAD is sudden death. And while the process may involve several office visits, I would contend it is better to know about CAD in the office and not autopsy. Agreed? With this assessment complete, you can exercise reassured the chest pressure you feel when running is not a heart attack. Several years ago, I volunteered to complete exercise stress testing to help train a group of resident physicians. Following the army protocol, my endpoint was not a target heart rate but sheer exhaustion. With chest heaving and heart pounding at 174 beats per minute, I gained confidence in my capacity and conditioning. On the outside chance CAD is discovered, it can be medically managed by addressing the specific factors that account for about 90% of the heart attack risk. If necessary, CAD can be treated directly with stenting or perhaps even coronary artery bypass grafting (CABG). Knowing about CAD gives you an opportunity to intervene; having CAD does not exclude you from the gym or the track. A structured exercise program, even after stenting or bypass grafting, is the standard of care.

The cardiac evaluation is the core, but not the complete, preflight inspection. Lance Armstrong's heart was tuned to perfection in 1996. Had he neglected to discuss the swelling in his testicle that October, the list of Tour de France winners would look remarkably different. There is no universal consensus on the scope of preparticipation exam for beyond-college-age males. Your age, symptoms, and concerns guide the balance of the process. Women have been conditioned from a young age to see their physician regularly. Men, not so much. As a group, we are reactive more than proactive when it comes to healthcare. Something needs to be obviously broken before we are willing to seek out a physician, otherwise, just rub a little dirt on it and keep playing. Usual sports physicals are framed in embarrassment: poking and prodding, then "turn your head and cough." Fair enough. At this particular opportunity, however, you need to voice concerns and articulate any symptoms. If nothing immediately comes to mind, the usual medical history forms and the symptom checklists can prompt your physician where to look. If you plead the Fifth Amendment and remain silent, your exam will not be accurate or complete. Despite the plethora of tests available, the medical history and physical examination remain the most valuable tools a doctor holds.

Aiding patients in understanding their health and helping them take steps to improve it is the chief responsibility of a physician. As an army aviator, I believed I was immune to the usual health issues of mere mortals until my flight surgeon pointed out high cholesterol. He gave some simple advice that I followed to the letter and kept flying. Doctors are taught, and the studies bear this out, that patients change their behavior at the direction of a physician.

Do not be surprised, or offended as I was, when you are asked about alcohol use. This is part of the standard package, not an accusation. Liver disease and cirrhosis cause only a small fraction of deaths in the United States, but intoxication accounts for about one-third of fatal falls, fatal burns, fatal drownings, and fatal poisonings.

I have had patients smirk during the screening for depression, but suicide ranked as the seventh leading cause of death in men in the United States in 2006, just below diabetes and right above pneumonia. Depression and alcohol screenings earn an A grade from the US Preventive Services Task Force; asking about them makes a difference.

If you are a smoker, your doctor should match his assistance to your motivation to quit. Presenting for a preparticipation physical, you have probably given it some thought. There are sprays, pills, patches, and gums to sustain your efforts. Anecdotally, I have found exercise to aid in quitting. If you are a smoker who starts to run, you will either quit smoking or quit running.

Patients regularly ask me, perhaps rhetorically, "Why can't I lose weight?" More often than not, the answer is eating too much, exercising too little, or both. Often, but not always. In my short medical career, I have diagnosed florid hypothyroidism in a patient who had put on significant weight over a just a few months. Basic labs, thyroid stimulating hormone (TSH) and thyroid hormones (T3 & T4), confirmed the diagnosis. The American Thyroid Association recommends checking thyroid function in men beginning at age thirty-five and every five years thereafter. This seems reasonable given the prevalence of hypothyroidism in the United States (eighteen cases per one thousand). Medications are another area to explore regarding weight. The list of prescription and over-the-counter medications with potential to add pounds runs from Abilify to Zyprexa and includes antihistamines, antidepressants, and antipsychotics. I can often scan a list and identify the usual suspects. Reviewing all of your medications with your doctor might lead to suitable replacement without the heavy side effect. Other conditions that cause weight gain, Cushing's syndrome for example, may have some characteristic physical findings that would lead to a detailed workup for confirmation.

The core of recommended preventative laboratory studies, fasting blood sugar and lipid profile, are completed with the cardiac evaluation. Based on your individual situation, after a complete review of your history and a physical examination, your doctor may want to order additional testing. Labs are easy to obtain, fairly inexpensive, and generally accurate. This begs the question: Why not order a full panel of tests on every patient? For the most part, random labs are a fishing expedition. They lead to unnecessary expense, unnecessary concern, and perhaps, an endless workup. Each laboratory study has a reference range of values, set by testing apparently healthy individuals. The 95% prediction interval assumes the values follow a normal distribution curve. Even healthy individuals have results that land in the high or low tail. Strictly by the numbers, we expect one in twenty results to fall outside the reference range, and there lies the danger of indiscriminate testing. An "abnormal" value requires a decision to explore, ignore, or retest. Exploration of a spurious result might lead to more blood work, imaging, or even a biopsy. I consider the standard army flight physical a comprehensive exam; the only two additional studies it mandates are hemoglobin (or hematocrit) and basic urinalysis. The first screens for anemia, the second for occult kidney and urinary tract conditions. There is no universal consensus on screening labs, and neither of the army's required tests I mention above is recommended for asymptomatic men by a national guideline. They are simply army requirements.

For a period of time, chest X-rays were a routine screening exam when the rate of tuberculosis was high, but this has since been discarded as useless. If you are a smoker or former smoker, a spiral chest CT has shown some value in the early detection of lung cancer, at a stage before it has spread and when it can be cured surgically. A few years back, full body CT scans were introduced as a proactive health screening tool. Other than the medical center selling the service, no one is recommending them. The radiation exposure is quite high, possibly provoking a malignancy down the road, and they have no real value. The scans rarely identify bona fide disease but do locate benign nodules, cysts, and such. An aviator I knew had the full body CT scan as he was "just curious." At fifty-five, he was healthy and active; the scan showed some stones in his gallbladder, a finding in about 20% of men his age. This incidental discovery immediately disqualified him from flying. He ended up having a cholecystectomy to stay on flight status. Curiosity was rewarded with an unnecessary surgical procedure. We both questioned the return on his "investment."

Any visit to the doctor would not be complete without some mention of testicles. They are the wellspring of testosterone and the core of our manhood. The testicular self-exam saved Lance Armstrong's life and should be completed at least monthly. Asking the doctor to identify any special lumps or bumps in your scrotum may feel quite awkward; most are normal, but ultrasound can sort them out. Underperforming testicles, hypogonadism, might be identified by marked atrophy, but the true measure is checking a serum testosterone level. Direct-to-consumer advertisements have raised the awareness of "Low T" and lowered the embarrassment factor. The initial screening testosterone level may be done at any time during the day. The second testosterone level should be drawn in the morning to confirm hypogonadism and would likely include free testosterone and steroid hormone-binding globulin, too. The

American College of Physicians does not recommend for or against routine hormone measurements. This should be a joint decision (no pun intended) with your doctor. The symptoms of low testosterone cover the spectrum from decreased sex drive to erectile dysfunction, irritability, depression, fatigue, and muscle loss. "Low T" can make losing weight more difficult. Any man from eighteen to eighty would have a potential reason to check a level. Testosterone is the end result of a complex process. If it's low, answering "Why?" involves more testing. Once the cause is identified, the question remains, "What to do?"

There are consensus guidelines regarding testosterone replacement and several methods of delivery including injections, gels, and patches. Testosterone therapy has been used as an adjunct for weight loss when hypogonadism is due to metabolic syndrome or body fat. Unfortunately, exogenous testosterone replacement suppresses the body's own natural endogenous production that might not resume for several months after replacement has stopped. Clomiphene, used principally for treating female infertility, has been trialed in men to treat erectile dysfunction that accompanies hypogonadism. Not so good for ED, but the researchers noted a substantial bump in serum testosterone levels at all ages. This has potential as a bridge therapy but is not commonly utilized. If testosterone replacement or clomiphene is employed, it need not be a lifelong commitment; reevaluation after weight loss is a fair strategy.

With the preparticipation exam out of the way, it is time to begin working out.

Hard Lesson #3: The number one cause of death for men in the United States is heart disease, primarily from modifiable risk factors. The preparticipation exam is the point to identify vulnerabilities early and intervene.

Homework Assignment #3—Schedule a Preparticipation Exam

Contact your doctor, let him know your plan, and schedule your exam. Ask about labs and the need to fast prior to your visit. Copy the checklist on the next page for discussion. Your necessary exam is between you and the doctor; it may contain more or less than what I have outlined based on clinical judgment.

Preparticipation Exam Checklist

☐ **Fasting Labs:**
    Lipid Panel (Cholesterol)
    Glucose

☐ **Review:**
    Family History (identify early deaths)
    Personal Medical History Regarding:
        Cholesterol
        Blood Sugar
        Blood Pressure
        Smoking

☐ **Physical Exam:**
    Head-to-Toe
    Focused Cardiac Evaluation

☐ **As Medically Indicated, Add:**
    Electrocardiogram (EKG)
        Exercise Stress Testing
            Echocardiogram
                Perfusion Studies
                    Angiography vs. CCTA

☐ **Consider:**
    Urinalysis
    Hemoglobin/Hematocrit
    Testosterone

☐ **Expect:**
    Depression & Alcohol Screenings
    Compliments on Starting a Program

CHAPTER 8

Left. Right. Repeat.

My life as a runner began in high school. Although the sports I chose did not specifically focus on running, each one used it as part of warm-up for practice. Our gymnastics coach required a loop from the gymnasium around the track and back, a half mile at the most. A teammate and I always added two extra laps just to show Coach our motivation. Training for my track event, pole-vaulting, required only short sprints. The first time I recall running any "distance" was for the USMC physical fitness test prior to enlistment. It was three miles long; it was hard. The marine recruiter pacing me from his car kept shouting, "Too slow!" and "Faster!" but there was little more velocity to extract. The run time was barely acceptable, and he strongly suggested training more with a casual "Boy, you better start running." I did not heed his advice and paid for it at boot camp. The penance was remarkably brief; my seventeen year-old body adapted readily to the daily rigors in the San Diego heat. Over the eleven weeks of summer, three miles shriveled from impossibly long to relatively short, and

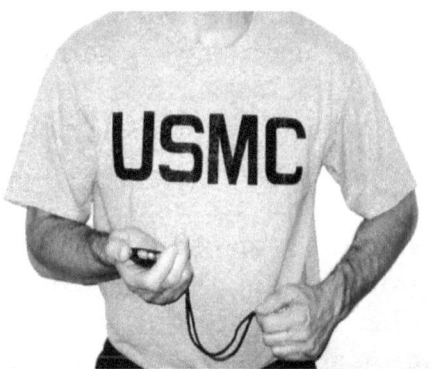

a six-miler became a solid run. Since then, endurance running has remained one of my primary fitness tools.

Humans are designed for endurance running; it is truly in our genes and expressed in our build. Fossil evidence suggests hominids have been running for two million years. Apes and other nonhuman primates lack the capability to scamper more than a few hundred yards. Human legs are long relative to body mass, giving an extended stride. Sturdy hamstrings rotate dense femurs across the hips' broad articular surfaces. Smallish feet keep inertia low, and tendons in the lower extremities have an elasticity that returns kinetic energy with every step. A narrow torso allows a slight twisting with each stride, the contralateral movement of our arms mimicking a quadruped's trot.

Our arboreal ancestors faced limited choices and quantities of food. Natural selection favored those who could travel. The ability to move quickly over long distances brought early man success in hunting and scavenging, success in the form of a diverse and protein-rich diet to feed a growing brain. Development of tools, spears, and arrows further sharpened our competitive edge. The profound human ability to create has altered our living environment exponentially over the past few hundred years. Rather than finding or chasing, we now grow our food stuff, even animals. The need to run down an injured deer has evaporated, nonetheless we still have the foundation. The DNA record shows our genes have not changed in the past forty thousand years and men remain genetically endowed for endurance running. A fundamental element of the Man Plan is exploiting this intrinsic capability.

The first step, literally, should not be the hardest. As a rule, men discontent with the trajectory of the FSL who hurdle into ten-mile runs risk catastrophic failure. Motivation failure and component failure. Our distant ancestors were walkers, and that is a fine place for men to start. Men walked for about 2.5 million years before we added endurance running to our skill set. Walking is a decent method of exercise, and physicians universally recommend it for some mighty good reasons, including convenience and very low injury rate. Leg length determines an ideal stride and cadence, lowering the energy cost of movement to rock bottom. Without instruction, men naturally fall into this pace, about three miles per hour (mph). A two-hundred-pound man walking one mile expends 106 calories in his effort, 318 calories per hour. At this rate, a man could walk forever and not break a sweat. Metabolically, the natural pace is pure efficiency. Yes, walking burns about 330% more calories than simply resting. On the other hand, so does mopping or washing the dog. Unfortunately, natural pace walking is an adequate program in the same spirit that "ten minutes of exercise is better than nothing."

For the Man Plan, we need more intensity. With a walking program, intensity is developed by stepping up the pace. Why move faster? A physicist might briefly argue that moving the load, your body, one mile by either strolling, walking, or running requires the same energy expenditure. There lies the difference between the physicist's definition of "work" (force applied over distance) and a layman's appreciation of "effort" (calories expended). Increasing walking speed above "ideal" ramps up the effort and boosts the calorie cost per mile materially. A higher speed requires a longer stride or faster cadence or both. At four miles per hour, the cost per mile has bumped to 114 calories, an 8% increase. Calories per hour jumps from 318 to 456, a 43% increase that reflects the higher effort over a longer distance. Walking fast is a relatively unnatural action; the fluid motion of the ideal pace is lost. The higher metabolic cost of speed is due in part to activation of stabilization muscles throughout the spine. The cost increase at five miles per hour is even more dramatic. There is some drama, too, just trying to walk five miles per hour. I find five miles per hour an uncomfortable walking pace, and it surprises me that race walkers can hit over nine miles per hour, faster than my usual running pace. To boost intensity without speed, adding a backpack or weighted vest increases costs proportionately but not nearly so much as speed. Intensity also climbs with adding inclines and hills. Walking hills at three miles per hour approximates four miles per hour on a level surface.

Walking	3 MPH	4 MPH	5 MPH
Calories/Mile	106	114	145
Calories/Hour	318	456	725
Estimates for a 200-Pound Man			

Speed multiplies metabolic cost and provides training intensity. Watch a man walking. You will note as walking speed increases, the movement transforms from natural to inelegant, inept, and inefficient. The body seeks tolerability, and this is unobtainable as arms flap and hips swivel artificially. Push even faster, and men change gears. Near five miles per hour, we instinctively break stride and begin running. This transition speed marks the point where running is physically more efficient. With walking, one foot remains in contact with the ground at all times. The back toe is pushing off as the front heel touches. In transition, the graceful pendulum movement of walking is supplanted by two springy pogo sticks. There is a brief airborne period where neither foot is on the ground. Regardless of speed, this is running. The metabolic cost of running five miles per hour and walking the same speed are identical. Above this speed, running is more efficient than walking—efficient in terms of calories per mile. Force a faster walk, and the cost of movement continues skyward. By transitioning to running, the cost of movement effectively levels off. Running, whether at five miles per hour or eight miles per hour, costs about the same per mile. Because of the longer distance covered, calories burned per hour continues to climb as running speed increases.

Running	5 MPH	6 MPH	7 MPH	8 MPH
Calories/Mile	145	151	149	153
Calories/Hour	725	907	1043	1225
Estimates for a 200-Pound Man				

Man is gifted with genes of a survivalist, the blueprint for a healthy, fertile life. Resourcefulness has given us a continuous supply of food and reduced demands for regular physical exertion to nil. The FSL is a natural consequence of this combination. Accompanying the life of leisure is the progressive erosion of manhood as testicles shrivel while infertility and erectile dysfunction emerge. Along with the belly and man boobs, we garner coronary artery disease, metabolic syndrome, diabetes, and early death. We are bright enough to understand the risks of the FSL and human enough to ignore them. Thrift is also a survival trait. Without predator or competitor forcing us to run, we relax. Though physical demands of life are reduced, time demands have compounded. Work, family, friends, TV, and sleep all compete for the precious hours of the day. Every facet of your life will argue against strapping on shoes and heading outdoors. This is the very moment when the Man Plan rubber literally meets the road. Once you take that first step, you are underway.

Through the years of medical school, running was an integral portion of my life. Before graduating, I had completed six long races. Two were standard length marathons, 26.2 miles; the remainder were ultramarathons, 50 kilometers or longer. I was a Runner. Residency training was a fitness thief as hours increased, stress mounted, and my selected exercise program consisted of sitting and eating. Marathoners talk about "hitting the Wall," a point in the run where they metabolically crumple and cannot continue, typically about twenty miles out. In 2004, I was thirty pounds overweight with deployment to Iraq looming when I started back running. On my very first run, it felt as if I could reach out and touch the "Wall." Immediately, I wanted to quit; this was the wrong decision. Yogi Berra remarked that "Baseball is ninety percent mental. The other half is physical." Your first run may be 100% mental. As no tiger is chasing you, the brain will rationally recommend stopping. Recognize this and keep going. With every shuffle, step, and stride, it gets better. Muscles learn the movements quickly while dormant metabolic machinery gears up for action.

The transition from fast walking to running can be eased with the walk-run. At the risk of oversimplification, begin your course with walking. After a minute or two, quicken your pace progressively until you break into a slow run. Keep running until your lungs or legs tell you to slow back, then walk some. Catch your breath. Recover. Step it up until you are running again. Repeat this process to your finish line.

Though I had previously been a long-distance runner, my initial program was twenty minutes through the neighborhood. Ten minutes out. Ten minutes back. That goal set itself. I had planned to go farther but red faced and panting, I turned for home at the corner. Total distance: 1.25 miles. Your initial goal depends on your conditioning, and the first few runs help you gauge this mark. I did the walk-run for a week, running longer, walking less, and each day moving out my turnaround point. Over the next few weeks, I extended the time from twenty minutes to thirty minutes. Within the month, running thirty minutes at seven miles per hour three or four times a week felt tolerable. The Man Plan is a whole life plan with getting started the biggest hurdle. It makes little difference in the long run whether your initial program is ten minutes or forty minutes. You are running.

The body is a magnificently responsive organism, and regular running induces remarkable changes rapidly. A six-miles-per-hour pace consumes calories ten times faster than just lying on the couch. Meeting this demand mandates aerobic (oxygen linked) combustion of glucose, glycogen, and fat. With the first strides, your body ramps up breathing and heart rate, multiplying capacity for oxygen delivery. It takes several minutes to warm up the process of extracting energy from storage. The first three to five minutes may actually feel more challenging than the midpoint of your run. This rest-to-run transition shortens significantly with training. More often than not, I start slow and advance speed as my breathing settles.

Regardless of your previous training, the first few runs or even walk-runs are quite a chore. Your body will move to accommodate the challenge as you push through this stage. Running several times a week compels a physical transformation in muscles and a conversion of fibers from glycolytic (burning glucose) to oxidative (burning fat). The density of capillaries, the smallest blood vessels, increases, improving oxygen delivery and lactate removal. Mitochondria, power plants of the muscle cells, increase in size and number and begin storing energy nearby in lipid droplets. A brave group of men allowed muscle biopsies before and after a sixteen-week running program. In this short window, oxidative capacity increased by nearly 20%, capillary density by 7%, and lipid storage by 21%. Neuromuscular learning, efficient fiber recruitment, and muscle memory improve run economy, and strides become automatic. Your body does all of this reflexively as it assumes you will be running again. If you resume the FSL, these magnificent changes fade and a former marathoner (me) can dissolve into a panting puddle after the first slow mile.

Through a series of interlinked adaptations, running is both restorative and sustaining for manliness. I call it "The Avalanche of Good." Muscles consume the majority of the body's glucose, commanding a constant supply with exertion. Running normalizes blood sugar levels as muscles gain an increased sensitivity to insulin. You might think appetite would increase to match your soaring energy expenditures, but a minor miracle occurs. In the early stages of training, only a fraction of the calories consumed in running are replaced by increased appetite. In one study, previously sedentary individuals were monitored as they trained for a half marathon. Over forty-four weeks, average daily intake increased by only one hundred calories. In sharp contrast, average daily metabolic expenditures increased by 30%. By my estimates, that is almost seven hundred calories per day for a two-hundred-pound man.

Men, unlike women, have no need to defend a certain body fat, and there is no hormonal signal to replace the "missing" fat. Regular running, even without conscious calorie restrictions, will lead to fat loss. This is how the army recruits and ordinary men get fit. The caloric deficit is preferentially supplied from visceral belly fat. With decreased visceral fat and improved insulin sensitivity, metabolic syndrome disappears and the risk of diabetes plunges. Endurance running serves to increase HDL (good) cholesterol and reduce LDL (bad) cholesterol. The heart muscle responds, too, improving pumping strength and efficiency. Running lowers systolic blood pressure and maintains vascular elasticity; both reduce the risk of CAD or sudden death from a heart attack. Whatever helps your heart helps your penis. Running not only protects the coronary arteries, it provides erection protection. Aerobic training facilitates arterial dilatation and improves blood flow. This is mediated by nitric oxide along the same chemical pathway affected by Viagra.

Running also activates the male hormonal axis, inspiring the testicles to produces more testosterone. After training only five weeks, testosterone levels measured in previously untrained men bumped up 17%. More important, their free testosterone levels jumped 26% due to the marked decrease in sex hormone-binding globulin (SHBG). The benefit peaks at moderate weekly mileage; runners logging over forty miles a week had testosterone levels drop though still remaining in the normal range. Reduced belly fat means testosterone stays active as less is converted to estrogen.

Growth hormone production, too, increases with regular training. Regardless of activity, growth hormone is released in small bursts over a twenty-four hour period with the largest fraction occurring during sleep. While the frequency remains the same, exercise increases the amount of each burst, and the total quantity released rises accordingly. Growth hormone was measured in men diagnosed with metabolic syndrome; high-intensity training bumped nighttime release by approximately 65%. Even low-intensity training boosted growth hormone release by nearly 50%. In sixteen weeks, the growth hormone effect on belly fat was apparent. Waist circumference dropped by two inches in the high-intensity group. More testosterone, healthy heart, less belly, and a firm penis. Can there be any more good news? Yes, runners logging less than fifty miles a week had improved bone density. The benefits begin when you do.

The United States maintains no compulsory fitness programs; running is a completely voluntary act. There lies the problem. Despite outstanding benefits that come on like an avalanche over a short matter of weeks, just getting started proves complicated for some men. There are a hundred perceived hoops to jump through including the embarrassment of that first run. When questioned, non-exercisers believed running took too much discipline, while runners noted the positive benefits. The majority of novice runners withdrawing from a half marathon training program cited time as the primary reason. Consistent runners made running a convenient activity with few, if any, lapses in their training schedule. That has been my success strategy. The course I run is handy. I change clothes at work and hit the trail on the way home. Hot, cold, rainy, windy, or even snowy, I still go. Former smokers return to cigarettes with just one puff. Runners can take the same fall by skipping training. Reading this far into the Man Plan demonstrates your intent. The challenge is translating your intent into action. Experts estimate it takes twenty-six weeks of regular training before exercise behaviors become embedded. I challenge you to start a program, any program, and continue it for six months.

Where to begin? Wherever you can. If you can only run once a week, then run once a week. Anything is better than nothing. A twelve-week study showed men running just one time a week made significant improvements in their aerobic fitness. Once-a-week training is far from ideal but can serve as your initial assault on the belly. In time, this thin end of the wedge may open up your schedule to something more substantial. Once the weekly run is firmly established, add more training days when you are able.

The running benefit is essentially dose dependent: more distance, to the largest degree, is better. From tracking the weekly distance and body weight of a sizeable group of runners, researchers noted that eight miles per week was sufficient to defeat the usual weight gain associated with aging. Twelve miles per week was better for fitness and body composition. Twenty miles per week was better still. The ideal running program early on seems to be three to four days per week, allowing the body time off to recover and adapt. Performance in a first marathon for a "low"-volume group training just four days per week matched the performance of a "high"-volume group running six days per week.

How hard to run is a fair question, too. Early in training, set the bar low and focus on completion. New runners are particularly vulnerable to volitional exhaustion long before any physiologic limit is breached. The brain accustomed to the FSL senses your effort and continually suggests stopping. If this happens, slow your pace, walk if necessary, recover, then start running again. Regular training reduces this mismatch between perceived and actual exertion. The initial goal is to establish running as a regular part of your life. If you are running with a partner, run at a pace that allows a conversation. This forces you to stay below the anaerobic threshold.

After the first few awkward weeks, when running starts getting easier, shift some focus to intensity. Humans have a maximal aerobic capacity (VO^2 max) comprised of genetic and training elements. Measuring this requires a sports laboratory, so more often than not, we use heart rate as a proxy. There are several formulas to calculate maximum heart rate; none are perfect, none are wildly inaccurate. The simplest formula: 220 minus your age. Intensity is expressed as a percent of

$$\text{Maximum Heart Rate} = 220 - \text{Age}$$

this maximum. For a man age forty, his calculated maximum heart rate would be 180 (220 - 40). Exercising at 60% intensity would translate to 108 beats per minute (180 x .6).

Target %	AGE			Intensity
	30	40	50	
	Heart Rate			
50	95	90	85	Light
60	114	108	102	Moderate
70	133	126	119	
80	152	144	136	Intense
90	171	162	153	Maximal
100	190	180	170	

Calculated maximum heart rate is a theoretical value subject to all the inaccuracies found in standard formulas. Use it as a tool to assess your effort. As your fitness level improves, your actual maximum heart rate (the upper limit) will increase. In short order, your running will become more efficient and the heart rate required to maintain a certain pace will drop, too. You will need to pick up the pace to maintain intensity. To track your heart rate on the fly, just lay your index finger atop your carotid artery and count the beats for ten seconds, then multiply by six. What a hassle! Instead, I recommend a heart rate monitor. They are inexpensive and accurate. Purchase one and wear it when you run. I was enlightened by this device, noting how much I can slack off on solo runs and how hot days really boost effort and heart rate. Using the formula, calculate your maximum heart rate and fix two numbers in your mind, 60% and 80%. Then get out and run. Ease into your natural pace and observe where your heart rate falls. Above 80%, slow down. If you are below 60%, just take note for now.

If I were to suggest a *target* program for a new runner, it would be: thirty to forty minutes, three to four days per week at 60-80% maximum heart rate (intensity). Perfect may not be possible, initially or ever. Start somewhere, anywhere. My initial runs were just twenty minutes. At the outset, the bulk of the effort is just adding running to your life. Once it is woven in, have a goal of increasing run time until you reach thirty to forty minutes. Aside from motivation failure, the biggest risk to a new runner is overtraining: going too far or too fast. The experts recommend adding no more than 10% in either time or distance per week. For persistent runners, the 10% rule makes sense, but for new runners, this rule is impossible to avoid violating. As you are starting out, rest and recovery should guide your training schedule. After any run, some soreness is expected. It may take one to three days, but you should be pain-free or nearly so before heading out again. If you ignore this, like I did, you may end up swimming for two months to allow plantar fasciitis to subside.

The training sequence should be initiation, integration, then intensity. The body responds rapidly, building, changing, and adapting. While there are obvious gains in days and weeks, it will likely take months

Initiation	Integration	Intensity
Day 1	→→→→	6 Months+

before you are ready to work on intensity. Again, this is a plan for life, not just the summer. Speed and distance will come with time if you have faith and just keep with it. New runners continue to make progress over the first six months of a program. At that point, after you have been sufficiently *imbued* with the spirit of running, it may be necessary to buy a good text like Noakes's *Lore of Running* to tweak your training.

The first days of running are likely to produce some aches. Shoes best suited for your foot type (length, width, arch, and pronation) can help minimize biomechanical stresses and overuse injuries. I shuddered when I read Jim Fixx's account of strapping on his old army boots and shuffling off. Despite this inauspicious start, he became a marathoner and the author of *The Complete Book of Running*. You

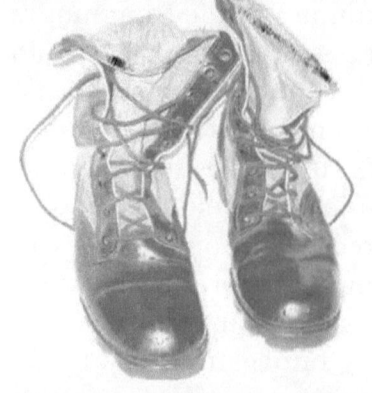

can certainly trial his method but, instead, I recommend visiting a running shoe store; let them know your training plan, get fitted, and buy a good pair. Consider this investment an inoculation against failure. Use these shoes only for running, and replace them every three to six months. When you are ready for new shoes, bring in your old ones for wear pattern analysis to further tune your next pair. Some specialty stores even have treadmills for stride analysis at low or no cost.

Nietzsche remarked, "There is more wisdom in your body than in your deepest philosophy." The core of a man's health is activity, sustained vigorous activity. I believe running is the most natural, efficient event a man can choose. Other endurance activities—swimming, cycling, rowing, and striding on treadmills, elliptical trainers, and stair steppers—are also suitable choices. The benefits of these alternates strongly overlap with running though they are less well studied. The event you choose should challenge your body with both intensity and duration. Running is clearly my favorite endurance activity, but I sprinkle in others throughout the month for some variety. Nonrunning activities may have certain other benefits, for example, no-impact striding on elliptical trainers. On most machines, the intensity level can be adjusted and many have built-in heart rate monitors.

Hard Lesson #4-Endurance training is critical to the Man Plan and the quickest, surest way to improve your health. Most men never get started, and their finish is predictably flabby and flaccid.

Homework Assignment #4—Hit the Road

Calculate your Maximum Heart Rate along with your 60% and 80% targets. Get fitted for new running shoes and buy a heart rate monitor. Choose your starting program with a goal of reaching thirty to forty minutes, three to four days per week at 60-80% intensity. Start running.

CHAPTER 9

Challenging Gravity

––––

The final phase of my medical training was a fifteen-month pain management fellowship at the University of Iowa. Each morning our small herd of doctors moved through the hospital on patient rounds, adjusting medications and infusions. The scope of our work, pain relief, did not limit us to any particular area of the hospital. We were likely to have patients scattered on each floor of the seven-story tower. My fellowship director, RQ, was a tall, gregarious Swede. On the mornings he led our group, elevators were forbidden, and we climbed the stairs. His efficient pattern of hospital rounds mandated beginning at the top, then working back down, floor by floor. He would lead a charge up the stairwell, literally leaping steps two at a time. Unfazed, he would watch the rest of the team emerge at the summit huffing and puffing, spent after just six floors of stairs. Early in my fellowship, before notice of my impending deployment to Iraq, this solitary climb was the sum total of my daily workout.

A few hundred thousand years ago, strength was patently necessary for survival. As we emerged from the forest, climbing a tree and carrying a kill were traded for tilling the soil and forging tools—still hard work. In the past few hundred years, machinery has supplanted this necessary brawn and essentially exempted men from a life of physical exertion. For the majority of American men, stair climbing might be the most physical challenging activity of their day, too. It takes a fair amount of leg strength to lift body weight in eight-inch increments up a floor of stairs against gravity. Walking involves a similar lift, though far smaller in magnitude. The body is raised only slightly by the legs and toes, then is allowed to swing forward and down. In reality, the core of human work occurs in opposition of gravity. The bones of the body have structurally adapted to counter this constant, pervasive force. Muscle strength, particularly in the legs, is maintained by working against it.

Remove this friendly foe and a man's body fades rapidly. Space flight is the extreme example of gravity's diminution. Without manufactured aerobic and resistance activities in orbit, astronauts begin to lose muscle mass immediately. Atrophy comes in the form of contractile protein loss over a matter of days. On a space flight seventeen days long, thigh muscles lost significant volume, about 8%. There was a corresponding 10% loss in power *in just seventeen days.* Without loading, bone structure suffers, too, and is directly related to the length of the mission. Over a large number of flights, researchers calculated bone loss in the legs and back at about 1% per month. Repair begins upon landing, but the process is exceptionally slow. Bone lost during a six-month mission might take three years to replace. The muscle and bone atrophy related to space flight have been compared to prolonged bed rest or immobility from spinal cord injury. The principle is clear: attenuate the effects of gravity and the body starts crumbling. This is not just a concern of a space shuttle crew. Once beyond high school, all men unintentionally acquire a pattern of avoiding gravity. More sitting. Less walking. Fewer stairs. With no challenging activities in sport or work, there is a progressive loss of muscle. Though the pace is much slower than experienced by astronauts, capacity and ability diminish steadily, and man is swept forward toward frailty.

Every week I see several patients consumed by inactivity and now reliant on scooters, stair lifts, and even chair lifts. The medical term for loss of skeletal muscle mass and strength is sarcopenia, roughly translated as "poverty of flesh" from Greek. Declining hormones and a sedentary lifestyle make it quite common in aging men. Common but not inevitable. Hippocrates, the father of medicine, observed, "That which is not used wastes away." This observation is still accurate today. Unused muscle is arguably unnecessary and, with the FSL, slowly, predictably evaporates over time. Sarcopenia is obvious in thin men; obesity conceals the loss, but heavy men become undermuscled, too. Between ages twenty and sixty, muscle mass in the ordinary male declines by about 40%. As muscle is lost, strength and work performance decline proportionately.

A further insult is fat. With obesity, it invariably infiltrates muscle, changing the texture and further eroding capacity. Intramuscular fat, known as "marbling" in the meat industry, is essential for a tasty rib eye steak, not a man's bicep.

Flaccid arms, sagging belly, and, finally, legs too weak to bear up body weight. Is this your destiny? Etched in every man's DNA is hope. We have held the same genes for the past forty thousand years, cultivated in an environment of physical adversity. Whether a man is eighteen or eight, he retains the capacity to build muscle. To engage this genetic machinery, a sufficient challenge is all that is necessary. Hippocrates also remarked, "That which is used develops." The defense against sarcopenia, maintaining and building muscle, is about challenging gravity.

Endurance running is work against gravity in micro-thin slices. With every stride, the muscles of the legs lift body weight just slightly and propel it forward as it falls back to Earth. There may be one thousand tiny lifts over the course of a mile run, requiring more grit than actual strength. Habitual running evokes a transformation in the muscle and its functional profile. Running multiplies the capacity to change glucose, glycogen, and fat into miles. Intramuscular lipid storage, oxidative (fat burning) enzymes, and mitochondrial density all increase dramatically. To deliver oxygen and remove lactate, miles and miles of capillaries develop. The constant, repetitive challenge effectively defers the effects of aging. Muscle testing, both macroscopically (peak torque) and microscopically (fiber area), of male master runners demonstrates the same characteristics of younger runners. For new exercisers, endurance running is an ideal entry point. Regular running devours calories, modulates appetite, and sheds pounds. The physical transformation over a few months is dramatic and self-reinforcing.

In the previous chapter and the above paragraph, I have extolled the value of running. My notion is this: a man limited by time and forced to choose a solitary activity to maintain his health and testicles should choose running. Endurance running unleashes a powerful force. Understand, however, the effect is body honing more so than body building. In a thirteen-week training course, though leg power of budding marathoners increased, muscle fibers actually decreased in size by 20%. As miles logged creeps past fifty per week, elements unnecessary for running are progressively polished away, even biceps. Arm circumference for ultra-distance runners is associated with race performance; smaller is better. High-mileage runners migrate to an unavoidably consistent body shape: skinny. At "fanatical" distances, eighty miles a week, even bones begin to thin, a suitable in vivo demonstration that man is engineered to be more than a distance runner. Running is the correct surgical tool to trim a man's body back to his foundation. The rebuilding plan forward is not more miles but a direct assault on gravity: weightlifting.

If you have never lifted weights, you have nothing to unlearn—a significant advantage over my errant experience. The lesson begins with some basic terminology.

- **Repetition**-Lifting and lowering a weight once.
- **Set**-A number of repetitions followed by a short break.
- **Load**-Amount of weight used.
- **Training Volume**-Product of Sets x Repetitions x Load.

All lifting programs rely on a pattern of sets and repetitions; you might see this written as three sets of ten repetitions or simply 3 x 10. Weightlifting strains muscles mechanically, damages them just a little, and stresses them metabolically. This is the recipe for change. How a muscle develops depends on where your program falls along the strength-endurance continuum. Quite obviously, lifting one pound five hundred times and lifting five hundred pounds one time produce different results though the training volume is technically and mathematically identical.

Running is an outlier on the strength-endurance continuum with repetitions likely in the thousands. Muscles asked to repeat the same small task *ad infinitum* develop the infrastructure (mitochondria, capillaries and such) as a response to the metabolic stress. At the opposite end of the spectrum is competitive power-lifting, where the goal is lifting exactly as much as you can only once. Building maximal muscle strength requires far fewer repetitions using a weight near the muscle's absolute capacity—a true physical assault on the muscles. At this end of the spectrum, muscles are injured from microtears and their response is repair and overbuilding muscle fibers. Moving closer to the center of the continuum produces the desired balance of strength, size, and endurance.

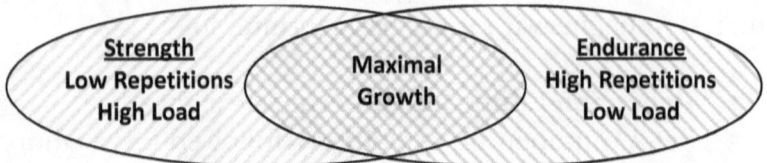

As an undergraduate in the 1980s, physical education was still a requirement, and I took the beginner's weight-lifting course. The instructor, a former football coach, was literally a huge inspiration with arms the size of my thighs. When I resumed lifting in 2004, like Jim Fixx and his ancient army boots, I simply picked up my old program, never considering what I had forgotten in twenty years or had never learned at all. I was defiantly self-confident about my knowledge, as doctors often are. The result was hours in the gym and scant progress. Somewhere along this interminable plateau, I engaged a trainer and simultaneously began sifting through research papers on exercise physiology. Almost immediately, there was stark realization that my understanding and application of lifting theory was horribly flawed. With a retooled program, I reengaged the gymnasium and began making progress almost immediately. Lack of progress had little to do with *what* I was lifting; it had everything to do with *how* I was lifting.

For certain, we have many more options in the gym than just twenty years ago. Bars with improved curves emerge each year, and weight machines add the elements of consistency and safety. Regardless of the mechanism, the process is just the same: moving a weight against gravity. Crucial to adding size and strength is continually challenging your muscles.

In college, Coach taught us a single lifting pattern, three sets of ten repetitions, 3 x 10. Applied to every exercise, the coach's dogmatic approach led to solid gains over a semester. The magic formula? Hardly. In reality, there is quite a range of programs that effectively produces muscle strength and size. A systematic review of lifting patterns revealed that six to twelve **repetitions** evokes the maximal growth response. This moderate number of repetitions builds sufficient mechanical tension to produce fiber growth and it causes sufficient metabolic stress to build infrastructure. The number of **sets** for maximal growth for the ordinary man is probably three or four. There remains some debate about the optimum number, but research clearly shows three sets produce more growth than one. Professional bodybuilders may use five or more sets. In practice, a higher number of sets is matched with lower reps and vice versa. A lifter might do three sets of twelve (3 x 12), four sets of nine (4 x 9), or six sets of six (6 x 6), thirty-six total repetitions in each pattern. The remaining variable is load. Higher repetitions (12 vs. 6) necessitate a marginally lower weight and produce more metabolic, perhaps even hypoxic, stress. Higher sets (6 vs. 3) give more rest and recovery time during the exercise, allowing more weight to be used. The resulting training volume for the 6 x 6 program is incrementally higher than the 3 x 12, but the value for the ordinary man is questionable, especially when time is a consideration.

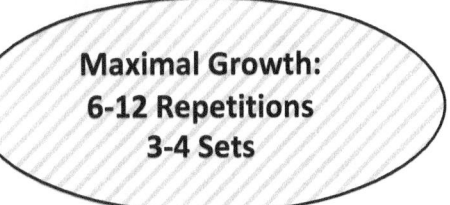

Maximal Growth:
6-12 Repetitions
3-4 Sets

How much weight to use is a trial and error process depending on the exercise and your fitness level. Something that pops up in many published studies and muscle building books is a curious quantity: the one repetition maximum (aka 1 rep max or 1RM). This is a tough number to find because it lies precisely between zero and two repetitions. Knowing this figure, researchers have some measure to assign training intensity. High intensity might equate to 90% of the 1RM; moderate intensity might equate to 70% of the 1RM. The proper technique for finding your one repetition maximum requires a trained spotter and, even so, might invite injury. I have never tried to determine a 1 rep max for any exercise I do. Curious, yes. Cautious, more so.

Instead, I recommend a well-constructed training principle: new lifters should start low and add slow. I could suggest that beginning light permits the muscles to learn the exercises and allows joints to limber. The truth is men are more likely to continue a lifting program when introduced with an initial low-exertion workout. Starting with one or two light sets of eight repetitions might not feel like much of a challenge, but recall the Man Plan is for a lifetime. In the initial weeks of your program, build to a full pattern: three or four sets. When you consistently push out all the repetitions, add more weight: 10% or less. Something I have faithfully (my wife would suggest obsessively) kept is a workout logbook, tracking exercises along with the weight used and repetitions completed. In a glance, I know if I should increase weight. A typical entry:

Exercise	Weight	Sets/Repetitions				
Bench Press	**175 lbs**	8	8	8	9	+

The final column is my plan for the next lifting day, in this case a "+" for adding more weight. Given my memory at times, the workout logbook is a must, and I recommend lifters keep one.

Turns out Coach did give us a decent starting program. In the initial weeks of *any* training program, neuromuscular learning and well-organized recruitment patterns develop. More efficient lifting allows adding weight rapidly. With regular lifting, muscle architecture remodeling can be observed in three weeks; an increase in muscle fiber cross-sectional area is apparent at six to seven weeks.

If a lifter continues a fixed pattern of reps, sets, and exercises, an inevitable plateau results. Consistently perform three sets of bench press, lifting one hundred pounds for ten repetitions, and you create a muscular system perfectly suited to lift one hundred pounds for ten repetitions, no more, no less. Invariability explains the genesis of my growth hiatus when I applied "3 x 10" over the long term. Perhaps Coach's game plan was to modify our sets, repetitions, and exercises in the advanced lifting course (had it been offered). As most weightlifting studies are completed over the course of a few months, the timing would have been about right. The ideal point to make a program change is shrouded in the haze. Some lifters change exercises every workout, employing a so-called "muscle confusion" technique. Others alternate heavy days (low reps/high weight) with light days (high reps/low weight). There is some comfort doing the same program over and over. Comfort but not growth. A conservative summary of the research would advocate a significant program change at least every twelve weeks. Shifting the elements (sets, repetitions, weight, exercises) renews the challenge for building bigger, stronger muscles.

Sustained Growth Requires Program Variations to Renew the Challenge

Another widely touted necessity for building big muscle is training to failure. During a lift, blood flow is temporarily constricted, allowing metabolic byproducts (lactate and hydrogen ions and others) to build within the muscle. This is a compelling stimulus for growth. In usual training (non-failure), a lifter might push out two sets of ten repetitions. On the third set, he pushes out as many reps as he can, maybe seven for example, then moves to the next exercise. In failure training, after pushing out seven repetitions in the third set, he would quickly reduce weight only slightly and do as many more repetitions as possible. Then quickly reduce weight again and push out a few more reps. Then quickly reduce weight again and so on. With no recovery time, the metabolic byproducts continue building, and ultimately pain and fatigue force the muscles to a complete halt.

	Usual	Failure	
	Repetitions		Weight
Set 1	10	10	100
Set 2	10	10	100
Set 3	7	7	100
Set 4	-	4	90
Set 5	-	3	80
Set 6	-	3	70

Some lifters express with absolute certainty that "The last rep is the only one that counts." That is just not true. Every repetition, not only the last, adds time under tension and applies metabolic stress. Multiple controlled studies show that while strength and size gains are identical, the potential for injury is much less with non-failure training. In a lifetime lifting plan, a few less repetitions are immaterial for growth whereas a shoulder strain might push you from the gym for weeks (or months or forever). Training to failure may also drive testosterone levels lower. In my book, this falls in the "Very Not Good" category, too.

Running for an hour is 60 minutes of continuous, vigorous motion. Lifting, in sharp contrast, is an intense but discontinuous effort. For several days, with a stopwatch I tracked the time required to complete twelve repetitions: it averaged 36 seconds. Considering I do three sets of eight exercises in a typical training session, my workout is just 864 seconds of actual pumping iron (about fourteen minutes). The balance of the hour consists of resting between sets, racking and un-racking weights, moving through the gym, searching on my iPod, and waiting on equipment. Muscle growth is strongly influenced by the rest between sets. A longer rest allows more recovery and allows using a higher weight. Powerlifters might take three to five minutes between sets. For maximal muscle growth, however, a shorter rest is better. Less rest ensures the recovery is incomplete and the metabolic stress continues ramping up.

Again there is a range to produce optimum results. After reviewing thirty-five studies, researchers settled on thirty to sixty seconds between sets as ideal for growth, this pattern producing the greatest acute elevations in growth hormone and testosterone. For me, a thirty- to sixty-second break is more than enough time to wipe away the sweat, log the lift, and take a sip of water. Extending rest by a minute would add fifteen minutes to my workout and more time away from home. I would gain nothing except a frown from my wife.

How often to lift depends upon your specific program and the time you have available. Ideally, a lifting day would be an additional workout, not a substitution for a run. If you can only lift once a week, then lift once a week. Anything is better than nothing (sounds exactly like my running recommendation). Muscles require recovery time to repair and grow. An initial program might have one or two exercises for each of the major muscle groups (chest, shoulders, back, legs, and arms). Allowing a day of rest between lifting sessions should be sufficient. When a training program becomes more intense, lifters tend to focus on just one or two muscle groups during the session but complete multiple exercises. Several days, or even a week, may be necessary for recovery. For my overall program, I have reserved about an hour a day for exercise and alternate running with lifting. Sixty minutes is sufficient time for me to do a five-minute warm up, eight different exercises, and finish with some ab work. The time commitment for your Man Plan has to strike a balance with the rest of your obligations.

Flaccid and frail are two words I never want written in my medical chart. Whether a man is heavy or light, without physically challenging activities, muscle evaporates through the years and sarcopenia is the predictable end result. Flaccid and frail. Weightlifting is an antidote for sarcopenia. Beyond building muscle, lifting has other exceptional health benefits. Just like running, lifting raises the level of growth hormone and testosterone. As muscles work more, insulin sensitivity improves, decreasing the risk of metabolic syndrome and diabetes. Arterial elasticity and cholesterol profile also improve, protecting the heart from coronary artery disease. Knowing all this, why would anyone fail to take action? Physicians, on average, live a little longer than most men. Is this because we have the full understanding and appreciation of the health consequences of the FSL? No, we simply smoke less. Doctors subscribe to the same adolescent personal fable of other men: "It won't happen to me." And then it does. I was fortunate to be spurred into action by the army. Over the past seven years, I have slowly recognized that shedding the FSL is not a zero sum game. The benefits far outweigh my time investment; there is no paired loss somewhere else in my life. Understanding is no substitute for action. However, in my case, it was probably the factor that replaced the transient external motivation supplied by the army to the continual internal motivation I have today. Most men are not fortunate enough to have an Iraq deployment looming and instead depend on erectile dysfunction or a heart attack to initiate their program.

As I close this chapter, you may note I have fully and completely avoided detailing a specific lifting routine. There are literally hundreds of suitable books to describe the various lifts and the muscles involved. A man can start a lifting program on the cheap in his garage with a bench and a basic weight set. My recommendation, however, is start in a gymnasium and engage a personal trainer. Together design your initial program, then put it into action. You will gain confidence in your technique and will make progress more quickly, reinforcing your Man Plan decision. The variety and quality of the equipment allow infinite variability as you develop your lifting program. Pay attention to the tenants of growth I have noted in this chapter, and always beware of the myths and miracles expressed as "truth." Though I look like a nerd carrying them around, my logbook and stopwatch keep me on track; I recommend using both. As I resumed my lifting program in 2004, I was wedded to a dogmatic program that quickly left me stranded on a plateau. Find yourself wedded to outcomes.

Hard Lesson #5-Muscle evaporates without use; the antidote is challenging gravity through weightlifting. Maximal growth is derived from the proper combination of sets, reps, and intensity. Limiting rest time between sets maximizes testosterone and growth hormone while reducing time in the gym. Lift hard but allow rest days for muscles to recover. Frequent variations in all aspects of a program are essential to avoid a plateau.

Homework Assignment # 5—Hit the Gym

Invest in yourself and join a gym. Meet with a personal trainer and establish your initial program, a whole body program using low weight and one or two sets initially. Start pumping iron.

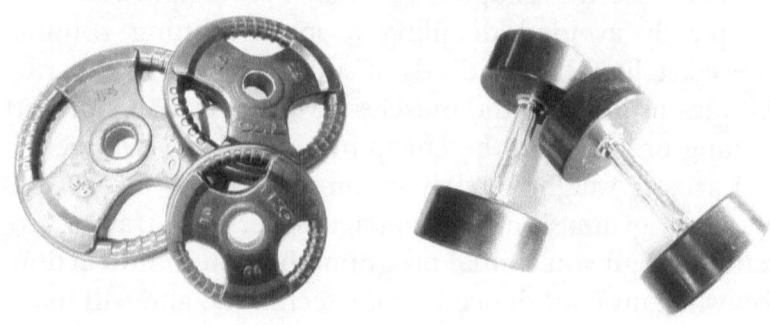

CHAPTER 10

Stoking the Furnace

The Man Plan is about building muscle and shedding fat: creating a positive protein balance while maintaining a negative calorie balance. Sounds complicated but the machinery of the plan is quite simple. In Chapter 6 I remarked army recruits improved fitness, lost fat, and gained muscle without any special instructions, just a lot more physical activity. This is the normal and expected outcome from devoting much of your waking hours to fitness training. For anyone other than a professional athlete, spending two or three hours a day in the gym would be impossible. Ordinary men have to mold exercise time into an already filled schedule. In a typical twenty-four-hour period, the average man spends about eight hours sleeping, six hours working, more than two hours watching television, and just twelve minutes exercising. I am committed to staying healthy but, nonetheless, limited to exercising just an hour a day. My work schedule cannot budge, but trading some TV time and a little sleep for biceps seems fair.

In the gym or on the trail, these sixty minutes have to be efficient with some incremental change every day. Paying attention to what and how I eat has made the world of difference in my progress. As we age, it becomes more difficult and then impossible to compensate for a poor diet, too many calories, and too much fat with a better (read: longer and more intense) exercise program. I see a Snickers bar and think: 271 calories, just over two miles of running. I can more easily skip the candy than spend another sixteen minutes on the trail. Applying this strategy finally got me off the mark in 2004 when I started a food diary and stopped eating a second breakfast at the hospital. Cutting calories alone leads to weight loss, however, in starvation mode, the body literally consumes itself. Muscle protein burnt for energy represents about 30% of the pounds lost—not a good long-term plan.

It seems counterintuitive that a man can lose fat and gain muscle at the same time. Old-school bodybuilders cycled through building and cutting phases. They pumped tons of iron and ate and ate and ate, creating the positive protein balance. The goal was adding on pounds of muscle with little concern about fat. Near competition time, calories got cut hard, but workouts continued unabated; excess fat evaporated in the process. Undoubtedly, they lost some muscle, too. A training cycle was months long, culminating in a contest. Healthwise, their program was pretty dangerous and not a sustainable long-term plan either. How can a man lose fat and gain muscle simultaneously? Simple: he can't. Ordinary men can follow the bodybuilder's training sequence, but the cycle is shortened to hours, not months. Within every twenty-four-hour day, there are building and cutting opportunities. Men have to create them and then apply leverage to the body's natural response. Not magic, just employing physiology research to exploit our genes.

There is constant protein turnover in the body with muscle breakdown and synthesis occurring simultaneously. A positive protein balance, more synthesis than breakdown, is muscle growth. Our ancestors were fully prepared for low-intensity activity all day long. Endurance training and weightlifting are exceptional engagement strategies for our forty-thousand-year-old genome. The actual fourteen minutes I struggle pushing iron or the hour I sweat running is sufficient to activate the same DNA. Recognize that exercise is only the stimulus for change; muscles do not grow in the gym. In fact, during a workout, breakdown exceeds synthesis and there is a small protein loss. Regarding growth, the hours spent outside the gym matter just as much as exercise; muscles only rebuild during rest and recovery times. The hormonal and chemical signals from a single workout may affect a man's body for two days. This is the window to apply dietary protein as our muscle-building lever. Protein ingestion, in and of itself, is a stimulus for muscle building. The proper protein diet will amplify the response to exercise, increasing area under the synthesis curve.

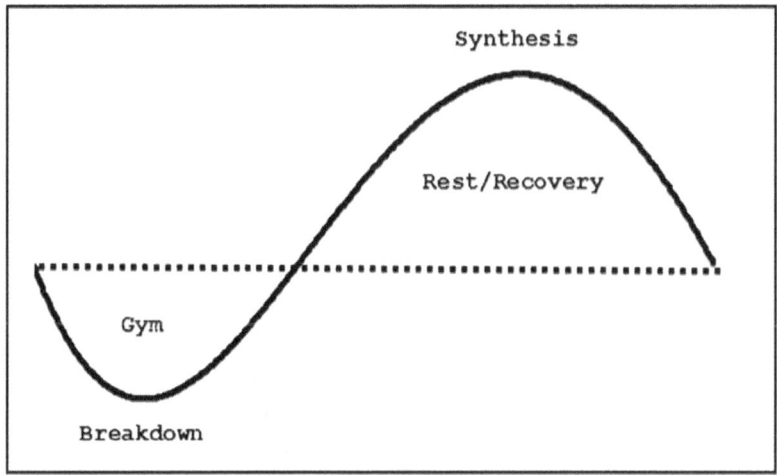

Most of the body's protein is maintained within skeletal muscle. Individual muscle cells contain about 16% protein by weight; around 70-75% of the cell is water. Man's proteins are built from twenty different amino acids. Some can be manufactured by the body, but nine "essential" amino acids must come from our diet. Digestion reduces food proteins to their amino acid building blocks.

The bottom line is you must eat protein to build muscle. How much to eat is a matter of continuing debate. Too little protein leads to a certain form of malnutrition, exemplified by the protuberant bellies and thin limbs we see in African relief advertising. Researchers conclude sedentary men need a minimum of 0.36 grams of protein per day for every pound of body weight. That would translate to 72 grams of protein for a two-hundred-pound man. Due to protein turnover and increased muscle synthesis, athletes need more, about 0.45 grams per pound just to *maintain* lean muscle mass. To gain muscle mass, they require an even higher dose. The American Dietetic Association recommends endurance- and strength-trained athletes boost protein intake to 0.5-0.8 grams per pound. A two-hundred-pound man intensely exercising would require 100 to 160 grams of protein per day.

Minimum	0.36 grams
Maintenance	0.45 grams
Maximum	0.5-0.8 grams

Bodybuilders, powerlifters, and other strength athletes may consume far more protein, but the advantage is not crystal clear. In measuring muscle protein synthesis, the benefit plateaus at 0.6 grams per pound for endurance runners and 0.8 grams per pound for strength athletes. This fairly well matches the American Dietetic Association recommendations. While too much protein is thought to be hard on the body, no one can state the absolute limit for safe protein intake. Studies conclude the maximum protein a 180-pound man can handle in twenty-four hours is about three hundred grams; deamination by the liver is the limiting factor. Just for perspective, three hundred grams of protein is more than two pounds of steak and more than 400% higher than the minimum recommended intake. Other studies demonstrate the body can only process about fifty grams of protein in one meal, a simple nine-ounce sirloin. Muscle building machinery, however, is max-imally stimulated by just twenty to thirty grams of protein. Strength athletes may have empirically discovered consum-ing excess protein keeps the muscle synthesis processes ful-ly saturated, but the goal of efficient muscle building can be met with far less protein.

Nearly all American men consume enough protein to sustain a sedentary life. The National Health and Nutrition Examination Survey (NHANES) noted that protein intake peaks in the twenty to twenty-nine age group at 105 grams per day, nearly enough to support an athletic life. Unfortu-nately, the distribution is not quite right for maximum mus-cle synthesis. About 20-30% of men skip breakfast entirely, a metabolic mistake for muscle building and fat loss. Tradi-tional breakfast eaters rely primarily on pastries, cereals, fruits, and dairy products, sufficient in calories but defi-cient in protein. Intake at lunch is generally better; an American dinner is typically protein overload.

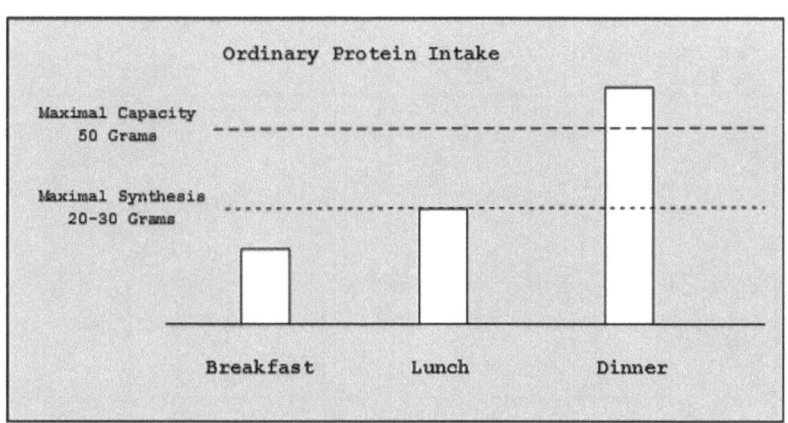

To synergize the Man Plan, we need to apply a little thought to protein intake. After eating, body begins digest-ing protein, releasing amino acids into circulation, pro-ducing a steep rise in muscle synthesis—perhaps 400% of the basal rate. Synthesis drops back to normal after a few hours despite a high level of amino acids still in circulation. Researchers infusing amino acids directly into the bloodstream noted the same pattern. Apparently, muscle cannot build continuously, and it takes time to restore synthesis capability. Eating protein constantly throughout the day is not an effective strategy, and eating just three meals a day wastes synthesis opportunities. To boil this down to a single point: a man needs five or six solid protein meals over the course of a day to maximize muscle building. If you allow that I am a strength athlete, my 160-pound frame would need about 130 grams of protein every day. Five servings of protein, about 30 grams each, would maximize my muscle building machinery. Breakfast, lunch, and dinner with two snacks during the day. This is no shortcut, just proper application of leverage, and the benefit is a progressive accretion of muscle. While the growth window after exercising extends for forty-eight hours, one critical period follows your workout. Always have a protein serving immediately after a workout.

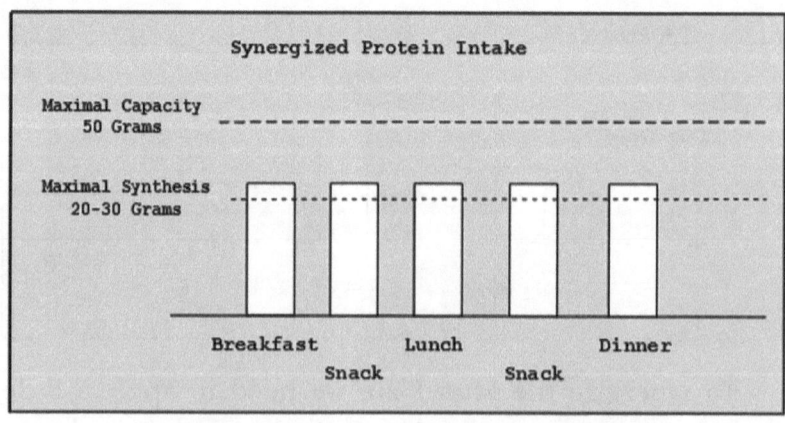

Even for nonathletes, five smaller "meals" a day is a good program. Eating more frequently reduces the rate of central obesity in men; the smaller servings are less likely to incite metabolic syndrome. Protein-rich foods have a high satiety index, satisfying hunger pangs and reducing unplanned grazing. Getting the right size protein serving requires reading food labels. Fairly quickly I gained a sense of protein content for my usual diet and learned that many of my favorite foods, bananas for example, were essentially devoid of protein.

30-Gram Protein Servings	
Steak	4-1/4 Ounces
Salmon	4-3/4 Ounces
Pork Loin	4 Ounces
Chicken Breast	3-1/2 Ounces
Red Beans	4-1/4 Cups
Greek Yogurt	2-1/2 Cups
Milk	3-3/4 Cups
Bacon	10 Slices
Eggs	5 Large
Banana	30 Medium

Following the Man Plan will likely involve changing many of your eating habits. Open up any health magazine and you are bound to be bombarded with advertisements for supplements. Looking at the claims and pictures, I ask myself: "Why don't I just try this magic muscle powder?" There are two underlying questions: Is it necessary? Is it effective? While we have understood the relationship of protein to muscle growth for years, sports nutrition is a relatively new science. Old-school bodybuilders relied on regular food—eggs, milk, and meat—to gain muscle. About sixty to seventy years ago, powdered milk and dried egg protein became available; weightlifters now had a convenient source of protein. While in college, I tried some "Massive Muscle" formula. I cannot say it made a difference as my overall diet plan was poor. It was expensive and came in two flavors: dirt and chalk. The flavors have since improved, and some are actually quite good. With emphasis, I will state there is absolutely no need to rely on supplements for protein. Are they necessary? No. Are they effective? Yes, but equivalent to the usual protein sources. On the other hand, it is not always convenient to have five scrambled eggs in your pocket. I drink a protein shake several times a week based on my work and workout schedule. Again, read the labels; most provide in excess of thirty grams of protein per serving. I use a half-serving of a particular brand, and it still gives thirty-two grams of protein when mixed with eight ounces of skim milk.

I stated earlier the Man Plan is about building muscle and shedding fat. Endurance training and weightlifting are complementary activities for this program. Endurance running burns big calories, and only a portion are replaced by increased intake. In sharp contrast, weightlifting does not burn a ton of calories. A two-hundred-pound man strength training for an hour (fourteen minutes of actual lifting) might burn 350-450 calories—far less than an hour of running (900+ calories). Research supports my personal observation: weightlifting boosts appetite, nearly 20% in one strength training study. This fully offsets any calories burnt and argues for splitting workouts into either strength or endurance days. Strength days can be calorie neutral while endurance days create a deficit and fat loss. Eating like a lifter every day allows muscle gains despite an overall negative calorie balance for the week.

An ordinary man may have five hundred grams of glycogen stored in his liver and muscles. This stored energy is readily available and enough for fifteen miles of hard running. Glycogen capacity only increases with training (and loading) and is the body's preferred energy supply during higher-intensity activity. At moderate-intensity running speeds, fat is the primary source of fuel. It would take over nine hundred miles of running to burn the fat off an average man. Even a 150-pound runner at a svelte 5% body fat has enough stores to cover nearly two hundred miles. Obviously, we have plenty of stored energy for running. What we lose along the trail is water. Strength athletes need to be fed; endurance athletes need to be watered.

The biggest component of a man is water, about 60%, with two-thirds contained within his cells. The remainder of body water is moving between cells or serving particular functions: cerebrospinal fluid, bile, and plasma for example. Water is lost continuously in normal body processes: perspiration, respiration, urination, and defecation. All through the day, water is sporadically replaced, primarily by drinking, though many foods have a significant water content. Unlike energy, man has no capacity to store water—a critical note for athletes. Some water loss is tolerable; men get marginally dehydrated on occasion during the day, and we grab a drink. Exercising muscles convert fuel to movement quite inefficiently, producing a tremendous amount of heat. Man relies primarily on the evaporative cooling via sweat for thermoregulation. Obviously sweating increases water loss, sometimes dramatically. Depending on the temperature and humidity, a two-hundred-pound man can sweat out more than two quarts an hour. To produce sweat, the body steals a little water from the intercellular space; blood gets a little thicker, and the heart pumps a little faster.

In physiology studies, water loss from sweating is most conveniently measured using body weight. A 1% loss of body weight in a two-hundred-pound man is just thirty ounces of water. Sweating profusely, two quarts an hour, this translates to twenty-nine minutes of running in the heat. With just 2% loss, about fifty-seven minutes down the trail, athletic performance begins to suffer. Heart rate has jumped, pushing a moderate-intensity run closer to maximal. At ninety minutes, water loss is over 3%, plasma volume has dropped more than 8%, and core body temperature is rising. Fully one-third of cardiac output is diverted to the skin for cooling. Performance is now down by 30%; the suffering athlete sags, then finally stops as the loss become uncompensable. Heat acclimatization improves the sweat profile and spares some electrolytes, but you cannot stop the water loss. On the other hand, the body has capacity to absorb water even on the run. The gut can take up more than a quart per hour—enough to offset a fair portion of the sweat losses. A runner regularly sipping water on a hot, humid day will not hit 3% loss for nearly four hours. On cooler days, runners can easily stay in fluid balance.

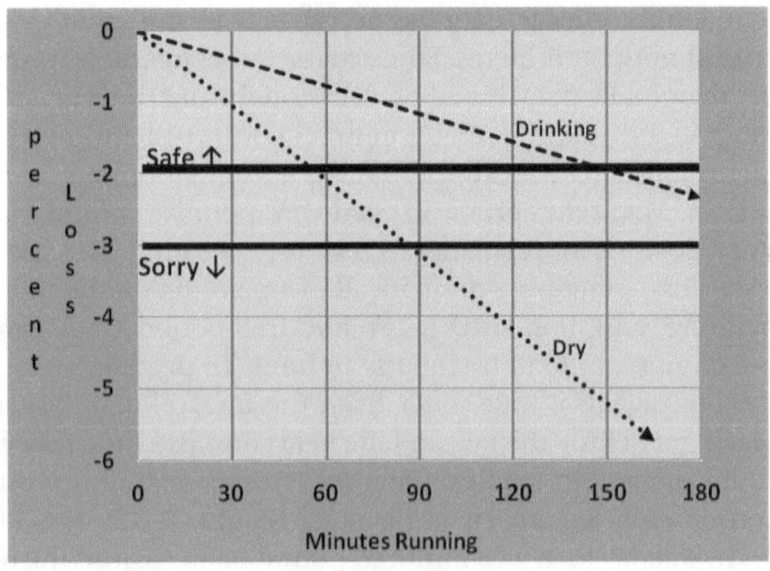

While my summer runs in Missouri are a hot, humid hour, it is impossible to hit 3% loss in sixty minutes. Based on my skin area, I just cannot sweat fast enough. Only rarely will water loss become a critical physiological factor for an ordinary man intelligently choosing to run in the cool of the day for twenty, thirty, or forty minutes. Then why have I even included this section? Any degree of dehydration raises heart rate, estimated at six beats per minute for every 1%. Any amount of water loss begins to erode performance, and how hard the run feels—the rating of perceived exertion (RPE)—begins to rise. Men not regularly exercising are more sensitive to exertion. For a man just starting out, a run may feel "hard" (RPE=15) at a heart rate some twenty beats slower than a frequent runner. Heat only makes it worse. Push perceived exertion too far beyond the comfort zone, and a new runner may mentally succumb. While there is plenty of physiological capacity to continue, he may stop for the day or perhaps forever. Starting out, we need to build the routine; the results will follow. An ordinary man, implementing a new exercise program, has only the sense of value of his plan. To keep with it, this value has to clearly outweigh any temporary physical discomfort. Hydration helps with comfort.

In college, I followed two rules while running: no rest stops and no water breaks. I believed both edicts tempered my soul and made me a stronger runner. Looking back, I wonder why I kept running. I take a short recovery break these days at key markers along the course and most always carry drinking water. Though thirty years older, I am able to run much farther and faster than I could in college. And I enjoy it. A proper hydration plan preserves motivation and keeps more fun in the run. The American College of Sports Medicine (ACSM) recommends prehydration before exertion and rehydration on long runs; the amount is based on weight and takes into account the heat. Following their guidelines, a two-hundred-pound man would prehydrate with fifteen to twenty-two ounces of fluid some hours before starting a race and, depending on the conditions, fourteen to twenty-seven ounces of fluid every hour during the competition. It takes some running experience to judge how much to drink in order to avoid dehydration but also over-consumption. On a very long, hot race, I watched my closest friend and running mentor retrieve a bottle from the trash. While we had been chugging Gatorade at every stop, sensibility interferes with even the best-laid plans. He rinsed it, then filled it from the cooler, only remarking, "I'm going to need this to finish." Sometimes, you just know.

For runs an hour or less, prehydration or rehydration on the fly is not physiologically mandatory; the benefit is essentially mental. Perception of effort, not absolute exhaustion, is an athlete's limit. Regardless of how far you are running, I recommend drinking fifteen to twenty ounces of fluid an hour or two before a run. My preferred beverage is Lime Diet Coke; caffeine gives a marginal boost to performance, too. Regardless of the temperature, carry something to drink. There are any number of suitable hand-carried bottles or waist belts. As the perceived exertion begins to climb, allow yourself a short break and a small sip, then continue on. Recovery breaks give the muscles a brief respite to mend aerobically. The major benefit, however, is psychological, splitting your run into several manageable sections. The challenge should be to your muscles, not your

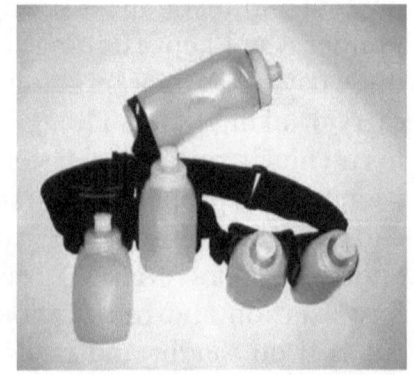

mind. As with weightlifting, an initial low-intensity running program increases the likelihood of it becoming habit. Resting and drinking along a run make it more tolerable, allowing a man to adhere to his nascent plans.

There is a lively debate about hydration with a sports drink over water. Clearly on extended runs or testing to voluntary exhaustion, drinks with sodium and carbohydrates improve performance. Along the average twenty- to sixty-minute training run, there is no physiological need to replace calories or electrolytes. If your goal is burning fat, science supports *not* consuming carbohydrates along a run. Lifting should strain muscle fibers; endurance running should strain their supply chain. The challenge in endurance running is getting to the point where the supply chain is actually challenged. Fluid or food carbohydrates can significantly reduce fat oxidation as your body relies on these new calories as a source of energy. That said, a twenty-ounce bottle of Gatorade is only 125 calories. If you need to get through your run, use it.

Hard Lesson #6-Weight loss without attention to protein intake leads to unwanted muscle loss. To maximize muscle synthesis, the quantity and timing of protein intake need to be tuned. Hydration and rest breaks keep the exertion at a manageable level, retaining fun in the run. This relative "comfort" is the key to initiating and integrating an exercise program into the rest of your life.

Homework Assignment #6—Stoke the furnace

Plot your day as a number of muscle-building windows. Based on your weight, calculate your daily protein needs (0.5–0.8 grams per pound) and divide this into five or six servings. Review your eating plan and transition to five or six solid protein servings (20-30 grams) per day. Meal, snack, meal, snack, meal (snack?). Ensure that a protein serving follows any workout. Prior to training, prehydrate with water or a zero-calorie drink (twelve to twenty ounces) an hour or two before starting. Find a suitable bottle or belt system for carrying water on the run, and plan for breaks along your route to rehydrate and recover.

CHAPTER 11

Beyond the Starting Line

———

There is a general understanding that exercise is good and belly fat is bad. True, but insufficient for motivation. Men follow an indecipherable valuation process in making any decision. The back story is very important. Accurate, complete information is a factor that can move a man from curiosity to contemplation to commitment. Indelicately, I have been ushering you to the starting line from the introduction. Specifically linking the FSL to progressive feminization, man boobs and fading erections, sets the stage. Consequences are another crucial factor. Psychologists understand the anticipated regret of a predictable outcome can guide men to an alternative ending. Someone frowning on the scale or cringing after his body fat measurement is primed to move. Many seize the regret, and the decision balance tips to starting a program. What advances a man to the starting line and what keeps him in the race are distinctly separate matters. New runners are prepared to suffer some in the beginning; however, the full cost cannot be appreciated until underway. Even with the best intentions and understanding, 70% or more bail out in the first six months.

Just prior to reporting to Fort Rucker, I took some private flight lessons to get a jump on learning. The classroom, preflight, and in-cockpit experiences were exasperating, an incessant reverberation of my ignorance. Throughout each session, the instructor would note the considerable gaps in my knowledge and skills with a comment or demonstration. Employing his training model, I could only fail. Invariably, I drove from the airport fearful I would wash out of flight school in the first weeks. Competence—zero. Confidence—zero. After a few lessons, I gave up in frustration and drove to Alabama with my gear and a lode of trepidation. The army program was remarkably different. The first flight in the aircraft, called the Nickel Ride, was a "no touch, just look" experience. The instructor pilots carefully paced the challenge of learning. Controls were added one at a time. I became competent to change altitude while he guided the aircraft, then I became capable in keeping the tail behind us at a hover. In a week, I could manage all the controls. After four weeks, I flew solo, then pinned on wings nine months later. Reflecting on the private lessons, it was method, not aptitude, that made the difference.

Physicians and psychologists spend careers studying patient behaviors in situations ranging from medication compliance to marathon training. Turns out the art of helping men change is far more complex than clever talk. Despite thousands of studies of sustainers and dropouts, it remains impossible to completely explain exercise adherence. Fear and regret provide the transient pressure sufficient to initiate a program. However, in the hierarchy of driving forces, extrinsic motivation is the lowest form. When this force fades in time, exercise declines, then stops, and returns to the margin. A consistent theme with "permanent" exercisers is recognition of value. Over time, extrinsic "have to" is substituted with intrinsic "want to" as the locus of control moves from external to internal. Central to this theory is sustaining until the profit of the effort is evident and the behavior becomes nearly automatic.

I anticipate most men will start with an endurance running program and add strength training later. Besides the low admission cost and near universal accessibility, the results are noticeable in weeks. The pages that follow are techniques of success culled from studies and experiences. Damon Runyon noted, "The race is not always to the swift, nor the battle to the strong, but that's how the smart money bets." Following these methods, a man is more apt to join the three in ten who maintain an exercise program.

Start Slowly. The perfect program is the one you can initiate and maintain. Anything is better than nothing. Granted, there is a dose response curve in exercise, however, the first several hours of exercise in any week are the most efficient in producing change. Even one workout a week delivers results in a man accustomed to the couch. Starting with a low-intensity program at the outset builds competence and improves adherence. The enjoyment-to-effort ratio will initially rest near zero, but the experience should not be overwhelming or defeating. If the summary of your first session is "That wasn't so bad," you have a better chance of running again. And again. And again. And again. Take the controls one at a time, focusing less on the effort and more on building the habit.

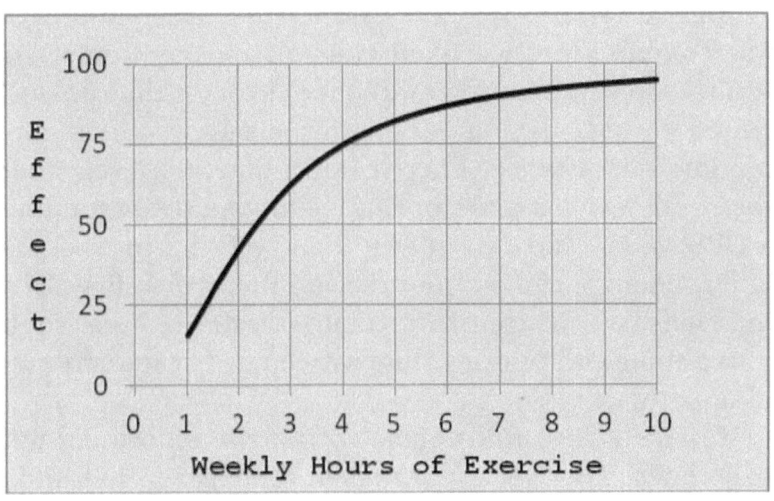

Add Slowly. Military recruits, transitioning from civilian to soldier, are plagued by overuse injuries from the abrupt increase in activity. Though the process is paced, for many it is still too much, too soon. Nearly 20% suffer an overuse injury; as a result some are held back in training, others are discharged. Experts continue to tout the 10% rule regarding increases in distance or intensity, and this is impossible to follow as a soldier or new runner. How do you go from running one day a week to two without violating it? Understand repetitive activity stresses muscles, tendons, and bones, setting off a chain of events leading to adaptations. For new runners, recovery is the real issue. With sufficient recovery time, the reworked tissue is able to tolerate further loading without injury. After a training session, some soreness is expected; you should be pain free or nearly so before heading out again. This may take one to three days. Dean Karnazes and his exceptional conditioning can run a marathon every day. As an ordinary man and experienced runner, I take one day off after my usual run and at least two days after anything longer. Lifting days are interspersed between these endurance days.

Insert Variety. When I first started back training, I was content to run a fixed course from my home. For several weeks I plodded and, once through the run-walk days, I started pushing out the turn-around point and extending the distance. There came a time, however, when the route was just plain boring. Someone recommended a GPS watch, and this addition allowed me to track my mileage and speed without driving the course first. This inexpensive tool transformed my single, tedious route into a thousand options. The whole city became my running path.

Choice is a central theme in exercise enjoyment and adherence. There is also a human tendency to fall into a preferred (read: comfortable) exercise intensity. Running long and slow teaches your body how to run long and slow. This mode is good for burning calories, but not ideal for overall development. A solid running program should include usual days, fast days, slow days, and long days. Sprints and walks. Hills and flats. These variations keep the challenge fresh for both muscles and mind.

Keep Records. Success in the short term is a major determinant regarding maintenance of a new exercise program. In the early stages of a program, it may be impossible to assess progress with a bathroom scale. Weight may be deceptively stable as body fat drops, particularly with lifting programs. The homework in Chapter 5 established your baseline body composition; periodically (daily, weekly, monthly) you should re-measure. Research supports maintaining both food and exercise logs. It sounds a bit obsessive, but adherence and outcomes improve. In a large weight-loss study, the biggest losers could be predicted by their logbook: more entries correlated with more weight loss. In another study, men who monitored their progress daily completed more training sessions than those checking in weekly. Essentially, the notes are performance profiling, confirming program effectiveness or need to change. On the track or trail, note running times and distances. Sum your mileage for the week, and keep a tally of total miles run. With lifting, recording exercises, weights, sets, and reps keep you from wasting a day in the gym. Training plateaus are easier to spot and correct. It takes months for an exercise program to become habit. These logbooks make it real, providing a visual validation further reinforcing commitment.

Intention → Planning → Behavior → Habit

Set Goals. A man always needs to have a target. True in toilet training at age three, true in exercising at thirty-three. Men who set goals in exercise are apt to do better. About 70% of new exercisers who set goals stuck with a program. In contrast, 74% without them quit. Overarching aims like "get healthy" and "keep testicles" are fine ambitions but require dissection into actions. *Specific, measurable,* and even *difficult* are goal qualities that lead to higher performance. Goal-setting has less effect if men cannot gauge performance in relation to the goal. An *outcome* goal—lose ten pounds, for example—provides a yardstick to measure success. In 2009, the surgeon general recommended at least 150 minutes of moderate to intense exercise per week, a decent goal. Keep track of your running times, and you can meet this week by week. Adding a precise target—like "run fifteen miles a week"—adds an additional expectation of effort. Translating 150 minutes into "thirty minutes a day, five days per week" adds specificity and forms a better goal. Now you can measure success on a daily basis. Pedometers have improved success in weight-loss programs because the trivial technology gives an up-to-the-moment report toward walking ten thousand steps per day. Overall, *outcome* goals are respectable, but they do not cultivate interest in the activity. *Process* goals intrinsically related to the activity appear to be the best. Rather than pounds, time, or distance, a process goal might measure heart rate or speed. A GPS watch and heart rate monitor can give minute-by-minute feedback to a runner. When your goal is keeping your heart rate above 130 for thirty minutes or maintaining a six-mile per hour pace for forty minutes, you know continuously how you are faring. This is performance profiling in action. A six-week study working with new athletes had the process group outperforming the outcome group at both the three and six month follow-ups.

Avoid Lapse. The best schedule is firmly flexible. If work or home prevent you from having a particular pattern—Monday-Wednesday-Friday, for example—then stick with a goal of three workouts per week. Review your calendar and plan training accordingly. When traveling or vacationing, bring the gear. Decent hotels almost always have exercise rooms, and I have stayed at several with arrangements at local health clubs. Recovery time is necessary, but resting too much gives the body reason to start shedding unused muscle. A short, fourteen-day pause in a group of runners showed reduced capillary density and decreased time to exhaustion. Plasma volume also dropped, bumping maximum heart rate up and increasing perceived effort. Not quite starting over but close if you are just starting.

Beyond performance loss is the concern of complete program loss. While attrition related to skipping workouts is rarely directly examined, in one study I could locate, 40% of the participants never returned after a "break" in training. The early months of a program are about consistency and developing the exercise habit. Most experts expect this process to take six months; others confirm a program lapse after one year is uncommon. By this time the motivation is intrinsic.

Employ Convenience. When selecting a gym, many base the decision on cost and equipment. My suggestion to base choice primarily on location might seem a bit odd. The medical center where I work has a fully equipped gymnasium and heated pool. Eyes light up when I tell patients about this no-cost facility, but only rarely does one become a regular user. Part of the reason is convenience; the facility is not on their beaten path. No cost but no value either. There are few studies regarding exercise and convenience, more often, availability and access are cited as barriers. I have been tempted to poll the regular exercisers regarding their proximity to the medical center. My suspicion is the distance to attendance ratio would be lousy, fading rapidly to zero beyond the ten- to fifteen-minute range. Since 2004, I have consistently chosen the gym closest to my home or on my route to work. This minimizes conscious effort and eliminates a physical barrier. I have been

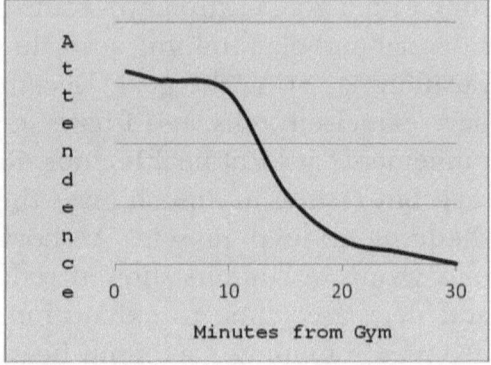

tempted to poll the members of my gym to discover how many reside or work within a ten-minute radius. The club's slogan "Getting here is half the battle" likely underestimates the true cost by 50%. For those tempted to focus solely on monthly membership fees, consider the cost per session. The "expensive" gym I attend four times a week costs about three dollars a visit. The "cheap" gym across town would save about one dollar a day while adding both time and gas expense.

Avoid Conflict. Every moment I spend at the gym is a moment I could be spending with my family. This is cost. Every moment I spend at the gym is two moments I gain in a longer, healthy life. This is value. With regard to exercise, spouses can be either patrons or critics. Following a heart attack or coronary artery bypass surgery, wives became active supporters of exercise and improved their husbands' adherence in cardiac rehabilitation programs. When the risk was only theoretical, prior to any cardiac event, spousal involvement led to early dropout. Immediate danger allowed wives to ignore the cost of a program; theoretical danger allowed them to ignore the value. I pull an hour out of my schedule every day to run or workout; my wife's consent and support are essential. A bright man will strive to keep the home cost low and the value high as he starts a program. Best as I can, the times I work out are de-conflicted with my family life. This means early morning runs while the rest of the house sleeps. I never miss my daughter's gymnastics, and exercise is never the reason we are late for church. I also hit the gym on the way home from work. This avoids the effort to disengage myself from the family. Timewise, it is exactly the same only different. A spouse who truly values exercise will work out, too, and that is the best family arrangement to promote adherence. Over a twelve-month program, only 6% of men quit a program when their spouse exercised versus 43% when they were solo.

Get Coached. A man can learn from reading, but one-on-one instruction promotes self-efficacy and builds confidence and competency. The gym is a busy place with hundreds of potential exercises. Unless you have been a professional gym rat in the past, employ a personal trainer for at least your first few sessions. This investment both demonstrates and raises your level of commitment. Even weekly meetings can move a contemplator to a sustainer. Aside from providing exercise instruction, trainers can assist with goal setting and lapse prevention. They also add the Hawthorne effect: men act differently when they are being observed. With a trainer watching, men push harder and move closer to their functional limits. Compared to unsupervised, self-directed exercisers, those assigned a trainer had better adherence (84%) and significant improvements in strength. Trainers vary across the board in education and quality. In addition to a supportive style and solid communication skills, the ideal trainer will have a four-year degree in an exercise science–related field and certification from a national organization (e.g., American College of Sports Medicine).

Try Racing. Running has been a part of my life for years, and I enjoy just getting out and doing it. In contrast, my closest friend always has a race on the horizon. His running program is about preparation: starting with a goal and training to spec. He garners T-shirts, medals, and belt buckles; I get "the best exerciser" award. Signing up reinforces commitment and adds some pressure to organize your schedule. Pinning a number to my singlet knocks at least a minute per mile off my pace. There is a race distance for every runner ranging from five kilometers to one hundred miles and beyond. Groups like Team-in-Training provide organized instruction and will send you to some exotic location for a race if you raising enough money for their charity.

Reduced Training. Men do not stop exercising because health has suddenly become unimportant. They stop because something else has become transiently more important. Life may intervene with even the best-laid plans, then a thought may pop into your head: "I need to hold up on the gym for a while." The Man Plan is not an all-or-nothing proposition. Athletes have off-seasons, and ordinary men get new jobs and more responsibilities. After my daughter was born, my program stopped for nearly two months. Starting back was starting over, rebuilding muscle, rebuilding habit. It does take a continuous, progressive effort to make continuous, progressive gains. This means always adding time or intensity to keep adding more muscle. On the other hand, maintaining gains requires far less effort. An analogous physics relationship is acceleration versus cruising. Trained runners logging fifty-plus miles per week were able to drop their distance by 70% without significantly impacting performance or power. When another group cut weekly mileage in half while simultaneously adding speed work, their performance improved. With strength training, muscles gain features not easily lost with detraining. A strength program can drop to once or twice weekly sessions without giving too much back. Lack of time is the most common reason men give for not exercising. When your time gets crunched, forget about stopping. Reduce your training only temporarily, and keep your gains and your manhood.

CHAPTER 12

Shackleton's Adventure

The title of this book was to be *The Tipping Point.* It opened with the negligible story of my rescue from a boat hull after Desert Storm. Sloppy sailing through the Persian Gulf placed me in an irrecoverable position: mast pointed toward the ocean bottom in waters teeming with jellyfish. Through my experience in medicine, I generally understood that FSL funnels men to a feminized frailty. I casually conceived a point-of-no-return for a man's health. At the proper combination of advancing age, inactivity, and increasing body fat, he would tip forever toward infirmity and thereafter lack the capacity to recover, à la my sailing tale. Through research, I sought to uncover, graph, and publish this "tipping point." It would have been a disappointing read for those discovering midway through they had already "tipped." Two things moved me from this title. First, as I painted the outline for my running partners, Jeff remarked the title was already in use. Thanks, Malcolm Gladwell. Second, I discovered almost immediately in digging through the published medical literature the tipping point did not exist. Regardless of age, regardless of weight, regardless of fitness, no man is ever hopeless.

With a corrected perspective, the tenor and tone of the story needed to change. Rather than a dark tome of impending failure, it metamorphosed into *The Man Plan,* a thinker's guide to escaping the mediocrity of the FSL. I pictured it as a lively but concise paperback a man could read sitting on the toilet and emerge with a strategy. A recurrent criticism of medicine is that knowledge held by physicians is shared poorly. The first few chapters of this book focus attention on the expected outcomes of the FSL and the underlying physiology for those changes. In a nutshell, we are so damn smart and so damn efficient, we have overwhelmed our ancient genes with calories and, at the same time, underwhelmed them with a soft life. And you now know as much as your doctor regarding why men get bellies and erectile dysfunction. The next several chapters map the path out of the woods, a basic how-to guide for avoiding heart attacks, man boobs, and ED. I have essentially expanded "Work out, eat right" and directed it to the sensibilities of adult males. And now you know more than your doctor about motivating your caveman genome. With this load of information, the playing field ought to be tipped in your favor.

Despite thousands of studies and billions of dollars spent, medicine has failed to defeat obesity. Certain small battles might be won, but the war is being lost. Our current solutions are as crude as leaches and bloodletting. Gastric bypass, a fairly effective tool for treating morbid obesity, shrinks the stomach surgically to a two-tablespoon-size pouch. The less invasive gastric banding places a coil around the upper stomach like a mechanical boa. Pills to regulate appetite, metabolism, or fat absorption have proven to be minimally effective, and many have been disastrous. Fen-Phen, a combination of fenfluramine and phentermine, was withdrawn after patients developed lung and heart valve problems. Meridia (sibutramine) had been on the market for over ten years. As data was gathered, it showed the rate of heart attacks and strokes went up in users. These medical "solutions" are well downstream of the central issue. Effective programs rely on increased activity and decreased caloric intake over the long term. Rather than chemicals or surgeries, thought and effort must be applied.

While the FSL should be respected as the most powerful erosive force acting on a man's life, it languishes behind the personal fable of invincibility. Unfortunately, as Aristotle remarked, "Men are swayed more by fear than by reverence." This was decidedly true in boot camp where my motivation to move was embodied in the drill instructor. Twenty-five years later, with an Iraq deployment looming, I had another concrete need to get fit. No debate, no choice, just action. Without a similar tangible motivating force, an ordinary man has to recognize and internalize the danger of the FSL from mere printed words. Early on, perhaps you were unclear about the extent of the problem or doubtful there was even a solution. In these final pages, there is no mystery why men gain weight. No mystery in the health consequences. No mystery how to avoid becoming feminine and flaccid. You may set this book aside, but you cannot un-ring the starting bell. With age and inactivity, the effects of the FSL move from theoretical to concrete, from never to now. Knowledge, however, is not equivalent to action.

Tigers have been around for nearly two million years and enjoy hunting, mating, and sleeping for the most part. Tigers do not get obese as it tends to interfere with two of their three favorite activities. They live concretely within their genetic jurisdiction, roaming the savanna, eating antelope, and drinking water. Men have learned to lounge in air-conditioning while wolfing Big Macs and guzzling Coke. A man can want Lance Armstrong's physique reflected in the mirror; the FSL ensures John Candy's brother will emerge. In the next one thousand years, it is unlikely that man's genes will transform adequately or our living environment will alter sufficiently so manliness is again the norm and health behaviors become instinctual. It is impossible for man to fully craft the harsh environment that hammered out his genome. We have to create it hour by hour in the gym or on the trail. And that is the rub of remaining a man.

The hurdle most men never clear is the very first; they never strap on the shoes and start running. Thomas Hobson was a stable owner in sixteenth-century England. If you wanted to hire a horse, you got the one in the first stall or no horse at all. His method was to protect the best animals from overuse. The option was simple: take it or leave it. A man without a plan is left with only Hobson's choice. While there appears to be a wide variety of options, in reality, you must either disengage the FSL or risk losing your manhood.

One researcher completed a diverse study of survivors, noting that only 10% knew instinctively what to do. Another 10% figured out what to do while the remaining 80% wallowed and waited waiting for rescue. Regarding the FSL, I wager *Man Plan* readers are part of the figuring group, the text only magnifying the nag they have already been feeling. Owning this book telegraphs intention. Intention leads to planning, followed by behavior, and finally habit. A recruiting poster for the remarkable 1914 Endurance Expedition reportedly read:

> *Men wanted: For hazardous journey. Small wages, bitter cold, long months of complete darkness, constant danger, safe return doubtful. Honor and recognition in case of success. Sir Ernest Shackleton.*

Twenty-eight men signed up, and twenty-eight heroes returned. Close this book and let your adventure begin.